Trouble Breathing

T0197969

McFarland Health Topics

Living with Multiple Chemical Sensitivity: Narratives of Coping. Gail McCormick. 2001

Graves' Disease: A Practical Guide. Elaine A. Moore with Lisa Moore. 2001

Autoimmune Diseases and Their Environmental Triggers. Elaine A. Moore. 2002

Hepatitis: Causes, Treatments and Resources. Elaine A. Moore. 2006

Arthritis: A Patient's Guide. Sharon E. Hohler. 2008

The Promise of Low Dose Naltrexone Therapy: Potential Benefits in Cancer, Autoimmune, Neurological and Infectious Disorders. Elaine A. Moore and Samantha Wilkinson. 2009

Understanding Multiple Chemical Sensitivity: Causes, Effects, Personal Experiences and Resources. Els Valkenburg. 2010

Type 2 Diabetes: Social and Scientific Origins, Medical Complications and Implications for Patients and Others. Andrew Kagan, M.D. 2010

The Amphetamine Debate: The Use of Adderall, Ritalin and Related Drugs for Behavior Modification, Neuroenhancement and Anti-Aging Purposes. Elaine A. Moore. 2011

CCSVI as the Cause of Multiple Sclerosis: The Science Behind the Controversial Theory. Marie A. Rhodes. 2011

Coping with Post-Traumatic Stress Disorder: A Guide for Families, 2d ed. Cheryl A. Roberts. 2011

Living with Insomnia: A Guide to Causes, Effects and Management, with Personal Accounts. Phyllis L. Brodsky and Allen Brodsky. 2011

Caregiver's Guide: Care for Yourself While You Care for Your Loved Ones. Sharon E. Hohler. 2012

You and Your Doctor: A Guide to a Healing Relationship, with Physicians' Insights. Tania Heller, M.D. 2012

Advances in Graves' Disease and Other Hyperthyroid Disorders. Elaine A. Moore with Lisa Marie Moore. 2013

Cancer, Autism and Their Epigenetic Roots. K. John Morrow, Jr. 2014

Living with Bipolar Disorder: A Handbook for Patients and Their Families. Karen R. Brock, M.D. 2014

Cannabis Extracts in Medicine: The Promise of Benefits in Seizure Disorders, Cancer and Other Conditions. Jeffrey Dach, M.D., Elaine A. Moore and Justin Kander. 2015

Managing Hypertension: Tools to Improve Health and Prevent Complications. Sandra A. Moulton. 2016

Mammography and Early Breast Cancer Detection: How Screening Saves Lives. Alan B. Hollingsworth, M.D. 2016

Living with HIV: A Patient's Guide, 2d ed. Mark Cichocki, RN. 2017

Central Sensitization and Sensitivity Syndromes: A Handbook for Coping. Amy Titani. 2017

Hurting Like Hell, Living with Gusto: My Battle with Chronic Pain. Victoria Stopp. 2017

Autogenic Training: A Mind-Body Approach to the Treatment of Chronic Pain Syndrome and Stress-Related Disorders, 3d ed. Micah R. Sadigh. 2019

Alzheimer's Disease and Infectious Causes: The Theory and Evidence. Elaine A. Moore. 2020

The American Cardiovascular Pandemic: A 100-Year History. David Gordon. 2021

Trouble Breathing: How Asthma and COPD Work and What You Can Do. Jeff Fraser. 2022

Trouble Breathing

*How Asthma and COPD Work
and What You Can Do*

JEFF FRASER

McFarland Health Topics

McFarland & Company, Inc., Publishers
Jefferson, North Carolina

ISBN (print) 978-1-4766-8610-3
ISBN (ebook) 978-1-4766-4498-1

LIBRARY OF CONGRESS AND BRITISH LIBRARY
CATALOGUING DATA ARE AVAILABLE

Library of Congress Control Number 2021052762

Front cover image © 2022 Shutterstock/Prostock-studio

Printed in the United States of America

*McFarland & Company, Inc., Publishers
Box 611, Jefferson, North Carolina 28640
www.mcfarlandpub.com*

Table of Contents

Acknowledgments — vi

Introduction — 1

1. Breathing—How's It Supposed to Work? — 5
2. What's the Difference Between COPD and Asthma? — 16
3. Isn't There a Pill for That? — 27
4. How Do I Take This Breathing Medicine? — 41
5. What Else Do I Need to Know About My Meds? — 56
6. What's the Deal with Oxygen? — 68
7. Will I Always Have to Haul This O_2 Tank Around with Me? — 77
8. Do I Have to Learn to Breathe All Over Again? — 87
9. How Can I Complete My Activities of Daily Living with Less Trouble? — 96
10. How Does What I Eat and Drink Affect My Breathing? — 105
11. How Can I Start an Exercise Program If I'm Having Trouble Breathing? — 118
12. Why Are They Doing Those Awful Things to Me in ICU? — 133
13. What About Other Common Breathing Problems? — 141
14. What About Other Non-Infectious Problems? — 156
15. Still Smoking After All These Years? — 167
16. How Can I Put This All Together and Make It Work? — 178

Glossary — 183

Index — 199

Acknowledgements

As easy as it was to discuss these subjects in front of an audience or at the bedside, committing these thoughts to the written word proved to be more challenging. I would like to thank all those at McFarland Publishing for their help with this project. In particular, Susan Kilby and Elaine Moore for their professional input and continued encouragement.

I would also like to thank Dr. Adam Griggs, D.O., for his initial review and clinical guidance as this project progressed. Thanks also to Ed Fluker, RRT, and Richard Hicks, RRT, for their administrative assistance which allowed our Pulmonary Rehabilitation program at Advent Health, Celebration, Florida, to mature and flourish. The success of this program would not have been possible without the dedication of my colleagues, Patty Ross, RRT, Dianne Anderson, RRT, and Gina Siberon, RRT. Skilled therapists whose enthusiasm, empathy and compassion fulfilled our mission to expand God's love by ministering to the body, mind and spirit.

And of course thanks to those many patients who participated in our program, whose determination to rise above physical limitations served as an inspiration to each and every one of us. Individual threads of life crossed here, each unique and colorful in their own right, carefully woven together by the hand of our Creator in a tapestry that radiates beauty and loving grace.

Introduction

Breathing. It's something we've been doing all our lives. In fact, it was one of the very first things we ever did and undoubtedly will be close to the last thing we do as well. Consider all those breaths in between, non-stop even while we're sleeping, automatically adjusting to ever-changing needs. It's something that doesn't have to be thought about—in fact, we don't—unless, of course, our breathing comes up short, and then it demands our immediate attention. Breathing is so fundamental to life that the brain is hardwired to warn us that when breathing is compromised, for any reason, nothing else matters. Survival is possible for a few days without food, water and even sleep, but not being able to breathe for even a minute will bring everything to a screeching halt.

Briefly getting a little out of breath is something all of us have experienced from time to time. Even while young and full of energy, we occasionally overextended ourselves and got out of breath. Fortunately, the brain immediately jumped in and told us to slow down a bit and take a few extra breaths. In a few seconds or so, things were resolved and we went on about our business. That was then and this is now. For the last few years, walking up a flight of stairs has been more noticeably difficult than it used to be. And recently those last few steps are a lot harder than the first few.

Until now, you've just chalked it up to getting older, but lately, even the simplest activity seems to cause breathlessness and it's getting frustrating. Those occasional asthma attacks seem to be more frequent, and coughing and wheezing have been constant companions. You now find yourself thinking about breathing more often and reevaluating doing things that were once taken for granted. Simple maintenance around the house, dusting, vacuuming or cutting the grass, is so taxing, the rest of the day is shot. A trip to the store now requires careful planning—*can't afford the extra steps if something is forgotten*. Dining out

1

in a restaurant? *Better not. Might start coughing again; what will peo-ple think?* Hobbies like woodworking have always brought joy, but now the sawdust is too much and the protective mask too restrictive, so the shop sits empty. And now this progressive shortness of breath has ele-vated your thoughts to the greatest fear: *What if I can't get my breath back at all?*

And that's the scary part of it all because shortness of breath is so devastating that you'll go to great lengths to keep it from ever happening again. But it does. Again and again. The natural inclination is to avoid doing those things that result in shortness of breath. Of course, now someone else has to pick up a larger share of those household tasks. And just sitting in the rocking chair seems to be the only recourse. If the stress of breathing weren't enough, comments like "You don't have any trouble sitting around all day but you can't even take the trash out" don't help either. We've always lived in a time where the doctor had a pill that would fix about anything, so we've never really had to worry about health matters. Now, however, the doctor has diagnosed chronic lung disease and ordered more prescriptions. And even with that, nothing seems to help very much. Avoiding shortness of breath while just sitting around waiting to get better seems to be the strategy, but things keep getting worse.

And therein lies the problem. The doctor can only guide medical management, but it's up to you to make it work—the doctor can't do it for you. In fact, survival is dependent on being an active participant with the doctor and not just a recipient of another batch of tests and prescriptions. To take the sugar coating off it: chronic lung disease is something one can either learn to live with or give up and die. It's essen-tially up to you. Simply taking the medicine as prescribed, hopefully, will bring temporary relief between episodes of breathlessness. How-ever, there's much more to it than that. And those responsibilities lie not with the doctor, but squarely with you.

When it comes to our health, all we want are answers, but because each of us is unique, there's no one-size-fits-all solution. Rather than simply listing recommendations or providing brief answers, I have explored the symptoms of breathlessness from various aspects. A better understanding of the questions that relate to breathing will allow you to have more beneficial discussions with the doctor to help fine-tune your individual medical care plan.

As a Registered Respiratory Therapist, I have worked in all aspects of cardiopulmonary medicine. I have learned from physicians, other therapists, nurses, pharmacists, and dietitians. But most of all I have learned from the patients whom I have had the privilege of caring for over the last 47 years. In order to more fully illustrate the discussion, I've highlighted the text with the actual experiences of others who have gone through exactly what you are now facing. I hope the information provided will help you become a better participant in your own health care.

1

Breathing—How's It Supposed to Work?

Shortness of breath for even a few minutes is an attention-getter. Fortunately, a quick recovery soon pushes that unpleasant memory aside. However, when breathing problems become more frequent, help is obviously needed. The doctor will examine, diagnose and prescribe an assortment of therapies which hopefully will help. Nevertheless, even with improvement, shortness of breath seems to repeatedly find a way to interrupt normal daily activities, which begs the question "What's going on here and is there more that can be done?" The short answer is yes, there's a lot more that can be done. The difference, though, is that the answer now lies on the other side of the doctor/patient equation; not with the doctor, but rather with the individual patient.

Searching for an answer without first understanding the question will be futile. Therefore, let's first of all review how breathing is designed to work. A better understanding of normal anatomy and physiology will be helpful. Although medical terms can be difficult, let's keep it simple. **Anatomy** simply means "where the parts are" and **physiology** means "what the parts do." When breathing is a problem, the lungs become the focal point of concern. However, the anatomy of the respiratory system has many more working parts. Physiological problems anywhere along the line can result in distressing symptoms such as shortness of breath. Let's start at the top and work our way down.

The nose: Actually the job of the nose is more important than just serving as a support for glasses or a way to smell what's for supper. The nose is designed as the designated place of entry for every inhaled breath. In fact, during the first few weeks of human life, nasal breathing is the only option. It is important to learn that the nose is for breathing and the mouth for eating. In fact, during the first few weeks of life, a stuffy nose can be a life-threatening problem. Fortunately for an adult, a stuffy nose, although irritating, usually isn't life-threatening. More than once I've seen patients in the emergency room suffer through a battery of tests because they told the triage nurse "I can't breathe" when in fact they just had a stuffy nose. The nose, however, is important in many other ways as it serves as the air conditioner for the lungs.

Incoming air is full of particles: dust, pollen, bacteria and viruses, just to name a few. Just look at all those tiny dust motes in the sunlight coming through the blinds. Unfortunately, the air outside isn't much better. Although the nose is well equipped to handle those tiny particles, it's the very small ones too small to be seen that often cause the most problems. The larger particles are usually stopped by our tiny nasal hairs before they even get to the lungs. This is the first line of defense in the process of cleaning the air and preventing problems further downstream. Some of those smaller particles are able to float past and would actually do more harm if not for a naturally secreted substance called **mucus** that lines all of the nasal passages.

However, mucus isn't just confined to the nose. In fact, every internal part of our body that air touches has a type of mucus-secreting membrane. Tears and earwax are a type of mucus. Tears actually have germ-killing properties, while earwax contains a substance to repel insects. Mucus is usually thought of as the result of an infection or the result of allergies. Actually, mucus is a naturally occurring substance without which our survival would be much more difficult. This slightly sticky watery substance traps the small particles as they float and tumble over it. Mechanically, it works similar to the flypaper commonly used in barns to catch flies. All tissues inside the body are very tender and sensitive to irritants, particles and fumes. The mucus secreted by the mucous membranes puts a bigger barrier between the irritant and those very tender membranes. This increased production also makes it easier to "wash out" the bad guys and keep them from causing more irritation or transmitting more little germs.

Most often, mucus is only noticed when we have an infection or during allergy season. When exposed to irritants the mucous membranes rapidly increase the production to wash the irritants away. After one handles something that could be covered with germs, running for an antibiotic isn't the first choice of action. Simply washing the hands is usually sufficient. And that's exactly what the body is doing. When there's excess nasal mucus, and sneezing or coughing is going on, it's the irritation that is causing the problem, not the mucus. The increased production of mucus—the body's "home remedy"—is just the body's attempt to reduce the irritation.

All too often the sinuses get all the blame. Actually, the sinus cavities don't produce that much mucus and don't normally get filled with mucus, in spite of what the decongestant commercials suggest. The sinuses have a very simple function: to lighten the weight of the head. If the head were solid bone, it would be too heavy to hold up, so there are extra holes called **sinus cavities** to lighten the load. Since air fills these spaces, mucus is also produced to coat the inside of the sinus cavity. A small opening in the lower portion of the sinuses allows drainage to the back of the throat. It's then swallowed in very small amounts that aren't even noticed. Sinus pressure occurs when the opening becomes plugged and the barometric pressure changes. The air trapped in the sinus cavity is unable to be equalized and results in a sinus headache. It's the exact same thing that causes discomfort of the inner ears when one is in an airplane: the inability to compensate for pressure changes.

The second important job of the nose is to warm each breath close to body temperature, which is normally around 98.6 degrees. For instance, if the inhaled air is 70 degrees, it needs to be warmed by almost 30 degrees in a very short amount of space. If the body's temperature varied by that much with each breath, survival would not be possible. Fortunately, the passageway from the nose to the back of the throat is not a smooth run. A series of four elongated and grooved spongy bones force the incoming air into a steady, regular flow pattern. The mucous membranes here have a shallow but rich blood supply that quickly and efficiently warms and filters the incoming air. The series of tissues resembles a conch seashell and is known as the **nasal concha**, or sometimes referred to as **turbinate**.

Anyone who has lived in colder climates knows all too well the instantaneous sharp chest pain following that first breath after stepping out of a warm kitchen into freezing temperatures. Unfortunately, all too often in colder climates we hear of a young, healthy person suffering a heart attack while shoveling wet, heavy snow. This is offered not to scare anyone but to illustrate how a better understanding of how the body works makes it easier to understand what can happen: The outside cold air needs to be warmed to body temperature and the diameter of the nose is just too small to allow an adequate flow of air. The work of shoveling increases the demand for more oxygen, and breathing through the nose and mouth become necessary. The inhaled air through the mouth is inadequately warmed and air passes more directly to the lungs. The heart is now working harder and demanding more blood flow. The coronary arteries, which supply blood to the heart muscle, lie near the surface of the heart. Cold temperatures slightly constrict the arteries, and as a result, blood supply to the heart is reduced. Unfortunately, the heart doesn't get the needed blood supply to meet the demands and the

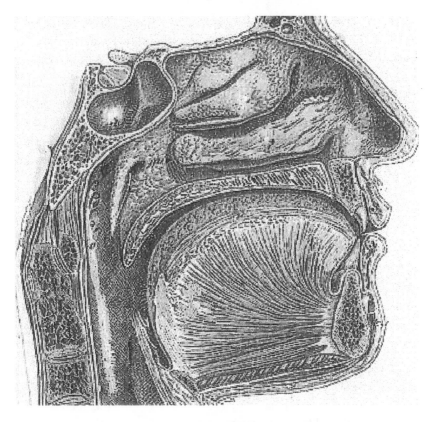

Nasal concha.

chances of a heart attack suddenly increase. This is just one example of how our body interacts with the environment.

The third function of the nose is to begin increasing the humidity of the inspired air. By the time the air reaches the first major branch of the airways, the incoming air must be fully saturated with water vapor. As air is inhaled and exhaled, the lungs and chest expand and contract. Things that are dry don't do that very well. The warm, moist mucus lining the airways moves moisture to the air passing over it. The moisture comes from bodily fluids that are replenished from the foods and fluids consumed. On a hot, muggy summer afternoon, that's not too much of a problem, but in an air-conditioned room the relative humidity is only about 60%. This means that an additional 40% relative humidity will need to be added to each breath. When the air is very dry, thirst will be more noticeable because more water vapor needs to be added to each breath. When one experiences shortness of breath, breathing naturally becomes deeper and faster. This will increase the amount of air needing to be processed and cause the mucus to be depleted of moisture faster. When too much moisture is pulled from the mucus, it becomes dryer and thicker, making it harder for any excess to be removed from the airways.

Down a little further, toward the back of the throat, is a common area where air from the nose can also be added to any air inhaled through the mouth. From here, the "air-conditioned" inspired air continues on down the back of the throat and flows through the **vocal cords**. They're located in an area called the **larynx**, which is also known as the **voice box**. When tilting the head back a little and placing several fingers about midway on the throat, vibrations can be felt when one is talking. The vocal cords don't normally affect breathing even if they become abnormally swollen and cause a hoarseness called **laryngitis**. The "raspy" voice is due to the swollen or thicker vocal cords resulting in a deeper pitch, much like that produced by the thicker strings of a guitar. Laryngitis usually goes away on its own if talking is limited for a day or so to give those vocal cords a rest.

Also in this area, at the base of the tongue, is the entrance to the **esophagus**. This is the tube that leads directly to the stomach. And right in front of the esophagus is the **trachea**, which is the tube that leads directly to the lungs. Swallowing normally occurs about 1,000 times each day without a problem. It's not possible to breathe and swallow at the same time, since the opening of the trachea and esophagus share a common area. Something needs to separate swallowed food from inhaled air. Fortunately, a small piece of tissue called the **epiglottis** efficiently serves this purpose. Given that breathing is more frequent than swallowing, the epiglottis normally remains upright to allow each breath to enter the lungs via the trachea. When swallowing, the tongue moves forward and pulls the larynx upward, causing the epiglottis to cover the entrance to the trachea. Now whatever is swallowed has only one place to go—down the esophagus. Notice how the Adam's apple moves up and down when you swallow? That's how it works.

While palpating the larynx a moment ago, you would have felt numerous individual rings. These are known as **tracheal rings** which surround the trachea and give it support to keep the trachea open during breathing. These slightly flexible rings are **cartilage**, which are similar to the material of the nose and ears. Since breathing is a series of alternating pressures within the airways, if there wasn't something to hold the airways open, the trachea would collapse. A vacuum cleaner hose has wire support to keep it from collapsing, and the cartilage in the trachea is there for the very same reason. The trachea is about 4 to 6 inches long in most adults and extends down to just behind the upper portion of the breastbone. Here the trachea takes two different directions (known as the **bifurcation**) to the right and left lung. The trachea is now known as the **right and left main stem bronchus**. The location and size of the heart cause the left bronchus to be angled more to the left, while the right bronchus has more of a downward angle. As a result, food or liquids that aren't properly swallowed often end up in the right lung; in medical terms this is known as **aspiration**.

Following the bifurcation, the airways continue to branch, much like the branches of a tree, and become progressively smaller in diameter. While looking at these progressively smaller breathing tubes it's easy to understand why the lungs are often referred to as the "pulmonary tree," a fitting description. These smaller branches are now too small to accommodate the thicker cartilage of the tracheal rings. Nevertheless, the function of holding these bronchioles open is still important. To achieve this need, the airways are now surrounded with thin bands of **smooth muscle fibers** embedded in the wall of the airways which hold them open. Although these bronchial tubes serve as pipes to channel air in and out of the lungs, they do a lot more than just that. Remember how the nose starts the process of warming, humidifying and filtering each breath? Although it does a pretty good job, air that is very cold, dusty or dry will be more than the nose can handle. Fortunately, lining all of these breathing tubes are specialized tissues called **goblet cells** that produce mucus. The exact same kind found in the nasal passages. The only difference now is there's a lot more of them. That's because the surface area of the lungs is substantially larger than that of the nasal passages. The total surface area of the nasal passages is about the size of a coffee table. By contrast, the surface area of the lungs is about the size of an average apartment. Every day, the lungs produce enough mucus to almost fill a drinking glass. A smoker, however, will produce several times that amount and usually have what's commonly called a "smoker's cough."

Although that's a lot of mucus, it's normally not even noticed. In addition to the goblet cells that line the walls of the bronchial tubes are specialized cells called **cilia**. More numerous than goblet cells, these tiny hair-like projections constantly sweep mucus upward to the back of the throat. The cilia beat in a very organized manner, similar to a swimmer's stroke. Pulling forward to sweep but then folding back on itself so as not to lose the forward motion. This effective escalator system will sweep mucus from deep in the lungs to the back of the throat in about 90 minutes. As a result of the trachea and esophagus sharing a common area, mucus from the lungs enters the esophagus and is swallowed. The stomach contains strong acids to help digest food, and, in this case, the acid effectively destroys any inhaled germs that are brought down. The swallowed mucus won't upset the stomach because the stomach lining is also being protected from acid with its own production of mucus. It should be noted that smoking significantly decreases the activity of the cilia. Even one cigarette will diminish the cilia activity for several hours. This is just one of several reasons why smokers cough more frequently.

With increased activity the cilia are stimulated to beat faster; however, as activity slows, less ventilation is needed so the cilia slow. Although the cilia are slowed during rest, the goblet cells continue to produce mucus at pretty much the same rate. In the morning, when first getting up and starting to move around, it's not uncommon for one to notice a few sneezes, runny nose and even the need to clear the throat of a little mucus. It's not allergies, just the cilia coming up to speed and sweeping up mucus that accumulated during the night. When one is admitted to a hospital or confined to bed rest, even for a few days, pneumonia is always a concern. In this case, pneumonia isn't something that is caught but rather a complication that develops. During bed rest, the cilia are slowed because of inactivity but the goblet cells continue to produce mucus. After a few days, the result is a "backlog" of mucus not adequately cleared from the airways. Gravity will tend to pull this backlog of mucus to lower in the lungs, resulting in pneumonia. That's why the nurses and respiratory therapists encourage their patients to get out of bed and start moving around as soon as possible. Those remaining on bed rest, are encouraged to cough frequently and take deep breaths to avoid congestion.

Farther on down, at the very end of the line, are structures called **alveoli**. Up till now, this has all been about plumbing, filtering and air-conditioning. However, at the alveoli is where it all comes together. These very small structures resemble bunches of grapes, and it requires the use of a microscope to really see them; they're that small. And small is what makes them so effective. An adult has around 300 million of these tiny air-filled structures, and surrounding each one is a network of blood vessels called **capillaries**. This is where the incoming air with **oxygen (O_2)** transfers from the air side of the alveoli, across that membrane into the blood, and the outgoing air containing **carbon dioxide (CO_2)** crosses back to the lungs and is exhaled. This exchange is known as **diffusion**. Impressive as is the size of the lungs, if all the tiny capillaries of the lungs were strung together, they would easily reach from New York to Miami.

The alveoli and capillary walls are very thin, which allows oxygen and carbon dioxide to easily move to the proper side due to diffusion. Earlier it was mentioned that differences in pressure were important factors in breathing. And in nature things go from areas of higher pressures (or concentrations) to areas of lower pressures (concentrations).

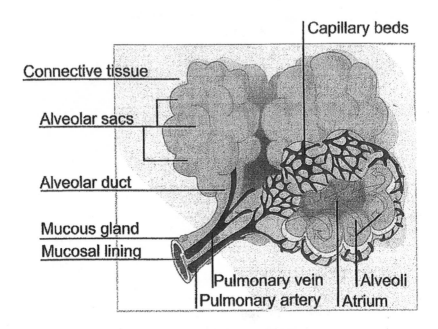

Alveolus.

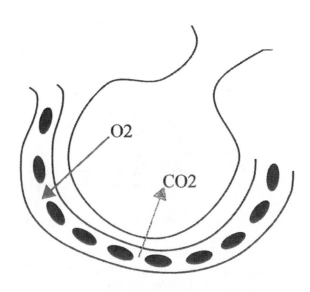

Diffusion of gases.

Just look at the weather forecast and notice how high-pressure systems flow toward areas of lower pressure. The inhaled air, which is now in the alveoli, has a greater concentration of oxygen and less carbon dioxide, while the capillary blood has less oxygen and more carbon dioxide. Given that the thin alveoli and capillary walls are all that separate these concentration differences, oxygen crosses into the blood while carbon dioxide crosses back into the alveoli. The oxygen that has now crossed into the blood is dissolved into the liquid portion of the blood. The dissolved oxygen now creates a **pressure gradient** that pushes the oxygen molecule onto the **red blood cells (RBCs)** which contains **hemoglobin** as well as **iron** to help to attract the oxygen. The oxygen is now **combined** with the hemoglobin of the RBCs to be transported throughout the body by the pumping action of the heart. When the blood flow reaches tissues that are in need of oxygen, the RBCs release the combined oxygen to the tissue because of pressure gradients; the exact opposite of what just happened in the alveoli. The cell now has the needed oxygen but it also has CO_2 that needs to be removed. Fortunately, since oxygen has just left the RBC, there's room for CO_2 to transfer back on the RBC and ride back to the lungs and be exhaled. When the RBC returns to the alveoli, the concentration differences reverse and the process starts all over again.

That's the trip through the pipes—the filtering, plumbing and air-conditioning units. However, just like the heating-cooling system in a house, the breathing system still needs something like a fan or bellows to get the air moving. The **diaphragm** very efficiently serves this purpose. It's a large curved muscle that separates the heart and lungs from the abdominal contents and extends front to back. In the resting position, prior to inhalation, the diaphragm is curved upward. At that point, the air pressure outside the body (**barometric pressure**) and in the airways is about the same, and nothing is moving. In order to make air move there must be a change in the pressure gradient to create airflow. Just prior to inhalation, the diaphragm contracts and is pulled down. The result is more room in the chest, and the air occupying this space now exerts less pressure than the air outside the body. A pressure gradient has been created so the higher air pressure outside the lungs has only one direction to flow, into the airways expanding and filling the lungs. During exhalation the chest recoils and the diaphragm relaxes and returns back up to its resting position. This reduced area in the lungs slightly compresses the remaining air so it flows out. There are a few other muscles between the ribs, shoulders and neck that are sometimes used for breathing and referred to as **accessory muscles of ventilation**. These muscles fatigue easily and are used mainly when one has

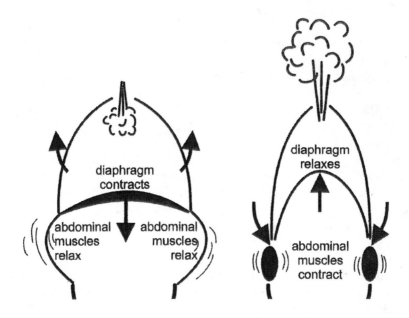

Muscles involved in forceful breathing in and out (Cruihne9).

become overexerted and is trying to catch one's breath. Fortunately, the diaphragm was built for the long haul and doesn't fatigue.

There's one other important component to this design that's perhaps the most important. Something needs to determine how much oxygen is required and how much needs to be exhaled in each breath. Just like any well-organized system, there are a couple sets of sensors located in a few blood vessels leading from the heart to the brain. The sensors are constantly monitoring levels of oxygen and carbon dioxide breath to breath, and sending this information to the brain for a response. As important as oxygen is to life, the brain is more interested in the levels of carbon dioxide as levels of oxygen play a backup role in regulating breathing. Two things concerning the stimulus to breathe are important to understand.

The first is that as energy is expended, carbon dioxide is produced and is one of the main **acids** produced in this process. In order to keep acids from becoming excessive, **buffers (bases)** are produced to maintain an acceptable range. This is known as an **acid/base balance**. The ratio is measured on a scale known as **pH** and the normal range is very narrow. As the carbon dioxide levels rise the pH falls and the brain is stimulated to increase breathing and reduce the elevated carbon dioxide levels. The opposite happens if the carbon dioxide decreases: the pH will increase and breathing will be slowed until the pH balance is corrected.

The second thing is that although the RBC will carry oxygen, the attraction for carbon dioxide is about 20 times stronger than for oxygen. If exhalation is not sufficient, more carbon dioxide will remain in the blood disrupting the acid/base balance. With additional carbon dioxide remaining bound to the RBC, less room will be available to carry oxygen. It's only natural to consider shortness of breath more closely related to inhalation; however, exhalation is of equal, if not greater, importance.

Medical concepts, physiology and chemistry can become rather complicated. It's amazing how similar these processes are to things used every day which seem logical in function. Consider an automobile. The amount of gasoline drawn from the gas tank must be proportional to the air pulled in through the carburetor to make the car run efficiently. Too much gas (rich) or too little (lean) and the car doesn't perform as it should. In a similar way, the body uses food along with a proper intake of oxygen in order to work. An improper intake of oxygen or nutrition and the body doesn't run as smoothly either. Following combustion, the automobile must exhaust its waste (carbon monoxide) gas, otherwise things come to a halt. Likewise, the pulmonary system must also exhaust its waste (carbon dioxide) for the same reason. Our faithful little car also requires routine maintenance to keep it running smoothly. And as the miles pile up, it begins to sputter, wobble and dribble a little more than when it was new. We don't think twice about doing preventive maintenance to keep it running smoothly. Unfortunately, many people only see the doctor when a health problem crops up. It's important to remember that one's body is not unlike one's car; as the years pile up a little more attention and routine maintenance is needed.

Perhaps by now it's becoming clear that shortness of breath is a bit more complicated than one might have imagined. It's easy to see why the doctor may be scratching their head when the chief complaint is "I can't catch my breath." A better understanding of how breathing is designed to function will provide the needed insight into why it's not. Let's turn the page and see what went wrong.

Additional Reading

"Effects of Barometric Pressure on the Pulmonary System," 18 March 2020, www.lecturio.com.

Kamashi Pandirajan, 27 April 2020, "Mechanics of Breathing," www.teachmephysiology.com.

Mariane Belleza, RN, 13 August 2018, "Respiratory System, Anatomy and Physiology," www.nurselabs.com/respiratory-system.

2

What's the Difference Between COPD and Asthma?

Now with a better understanding of how our breathing is designed to work, let's use that information to reconstruct what's wrong. Of course, the common complaint is "I can't breathe" and there very well may be lots of reasons why. As the old adage goes, "When one wheel comes loose on the wagon, they all start to wobble." And this is very true of the body. When one system is compromised, other systems try to take up the slack. Unfortunately, that can only last for so long before they start to be compromised as well. Fixing the immediate problem is of course the first priority, but the bigger question ... what caused it?

Before going any farther, a few more medical terms need to be introduced. The first pair are the terms **acute** and **chronic**. "Acute" refers to a problem that's of a recent nature and is likely to resolve itself shortly. A cold or the flu are common examples of an acute infection. "Chronic," on the other hand, indicates a problem of a more long-standing nature— unfortunately, one not likely to be resolved for a while, if ever. The next term isn't a word but rather the suffix **-itis**, which refers to inflammation or swelling. Combining this suffix with an anatomical part describes what is happening and where. For instance, **bronchitis** means that the bronchial tubes are inflamed. An episode of acute bronchitis can occur when one is afflicted with a cold or the flu. The bronchial tubes are inflamed but return to normal in a week or so. The reason the inflammation goes away is that an acute **upper respiratory infection (URI)** is the result of exposure to an irritating substance such as a germ. The symptoms will likely disappear due to the shorter life cycle of those germs or when the irritating substance is gone. With the irritation gone, the bronchial tubes won't need to keep producing excessive mucus for protection. However, if the cause is prolonged, with years of constant irritation and inflammation, the airways will undergo a process called **remodeling**. This essentially is the body's attempt to adapt and lessen the effects of the persistent irritation. Two changes begin to happen: In order to stabilize the smaller bronchial tubes, the walls begin to thicken. Unfortunately, the thickening occurs within the walls, decreasing the diameter that air has to flow through. Also, the mucus-producing goblet cells eventually enlarge to keep up with the demand. The thicker layer of mucus provides an increased barrier between the irritant and the delicate bronchial walls. As a result, the thickened walls of the airways combined with the extra mucus further slow the movement of air. This slowing of airflow is termed **increased resistance** and breathing becomes more difficult. Frequent coughing, in order to clear the airways, becomes a normal part of one's routine. Unfortunately, following remodeling, if the irritation is no longer there, the airways aren't likely to revert back to normal. The enlarged goblet cells continue to produce excessive mucus and airflow is partially obstructed. This condition is now termed a "chronic bronchitis," one that's been coming about for quite a while and not likely to go away anytime soon ... if ever. Anyone who has been a cigarette smoker for a significant amount of time and has a "smoker's cough" is likely to have chronic bronchitis. Smoking, however, isn't the only cause. Many environmental service workers who have never smoked develop chronic bronchitis after years of inhaling the caustic fumes of cleaning solutions. And that leads us to a more serious discussion.

COPD: **Chronic bronchitis** and **emphysema** are the two diseases that come under the umbrella known as COPD, which stands for

Chronic Obstructive Pulmonary Disease

Chronic means it's been going on for a considerable amount of time.

Obstructive means that air isn't flowing freely through the airways.

P stands for pulmonary, which refers to the lungs.

D stands for disease, meaning this just isn't normal.

Although a disease is often thought of as something that is caught, neither chronic bronchitis nor emphysema can be caught. Let's take a look at these two problems and how they're similar and yet different.

Chronic bronchitis is a condition diagnosed by history. The generally accepted guidelines are a history of a productive cough for at least three months during the last two consecutive years. An active infection may or may not be going on. The excessive mucus is the normal response

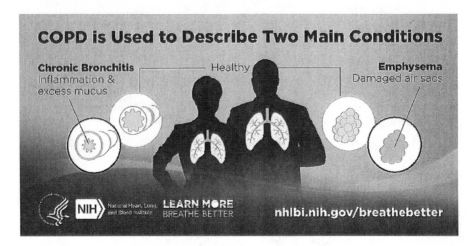

COPD.

to prolonged irritation of the bronchial tubes. Once remodeling has taken place, excessive mucus will become the new normal. This process is usually gradual, and frequent coughing has become part of the daily routine and not really noticed. Middle-aged adults are more often diagnosed with chronic bronchitis when other symptoms such as excessive fatigue, weakness and dizziness begin to interfere with work or social activities. However, since the excessive airway mucus is warm, moist and appealing to any inhaled bacteria or virus, frequent URIs are more likely to necessitate medical intervention rather than the cough alone. Diagnosis is typically based on a medical exam and a history of smoking as well as occupational and environmental exposures. Physical and laboratory exams will also be needed to rule out other causes. Although medications will likely be prescribed, they will only temporarily relieve the symptoms. More importantly, though, unless the cause of the irritation is removed the problems will soon return and continue to get worse.

With *emphysema*, the other disease classified as COPD, the problem is with the alveoli where the gases are exchanged with the blood. The alveoli are very thin, elastic tissue that expand and partially deflate with each breath. The gas exchange in the alveoli is so efficient because of their extremely small size. Yet they comprise a surface area of about 750 square feet, and it's this extremely large surface area that makes breathing so efficient. With emphysema, many of the alveoli walls have deteriorated into larger pockets. Unfortunately, in this case, bigger is not better. Fewer but larger alveoli actually reduce the total surface area that millions of smaller alveoli normally provide. The result is less available area to exchange oxygen and carbon dioxide with the blood.

Unfortunately, there's a little more to it than just that. To better visualize the problem, let's imagine here that a single alveolus is like a brand-new balloon. When it's first blown up, it takes a lot of pressure, but the second time it's not quite so difficult. That's because it has been partially stretched. Because of this stretching, when the air from the balloon is released, the balloon doesn't quite go back to its original shape. The alveoli work about the same way as that balloon; they inflate and partially deflate with each breath. A small amount of air remains behind to keep the alveoli from collapsing. This is called the **residual volume** and helps the alveoli to re-inflate. The residual volume retains a higher percentage of carbon dioxide and mixes with the incoming air that has a higher percentage of oxygen. With emphysema, the abnormally enlarged alveoli retain a larger amount of un-exhaled residual air. Although the red blood cells are waiting to be loaded with oxygen, carbon dioxide is bound about 20 times more tightly to the RBCs. The net result is less room for oxygen to be carried by the RBCs.

The obstruction portion of emphysema occurs because, although the alveoli became larger, the **terminal bronchiole**, where it enters the alveoli, remained about the same diameter. That means that the larger volume of residual air waiting to be exhaled is more than can fit back through the terminal bronchiole. This obstruction during exhalation is responsible for the larger amount of trapped (residual) air. Picture the day after Thanksgiving with 500 shoppers trying to go through the same door at the same time. Things just get jammed up at the door. If you're trying to explain this to someone who doesn't understand what you're going through, have them try this: take in a normal breath but only exhale half of it. Now inhale again and only exhale half of that breath as well. After just a few times, they'll be rushing to fully exhale. They will quickly understand what you're going through. The partial obstruction of that exhaled air is fundamental to shortness of breath, and we'll find some solutions to the problem in subsequent chapters.

Unfortunately, difficulty exhaling isn't the only problem with COPD because the ability to inhale is compromised as well. As noted, the diaphragm, just prior to inhalation, is dome shaped. During inhalation, it is pulled downward to create a pressure change and allow air to flow into the lungs. With emphysema, those enlarged air-filled alveoli are occupying more area in the chest than they should. This is known as **hyperinflation**, meaning the alveoli are holding a larger volume of air than they were designed to hold. In view of the fact that the chest cavity has a limited amount of room, something's got to give. Ribs hold the chest in place so outward expansion is limited. Bones that anchor the shoulders (collarbones) limit the ability to expand upward. So, the only direction left is downward, pressing on the diaphragm, causing it to be more flattened. The ability to inhale is still dependent on pressure differences, but since the diaphragm has lost much of its dome shape, movement is limited. In order to move an adequate amount of air, breathing becomes shallow and more rapid (**hyperventilation**). In an attempt to compensate for the reduced diaphragmatic movement, muscles in the upper chest, neck, and between the ribs are used to pull the chest up and outward. Even minor exertions or position changes frequently result in shortness of breath. Recovery is slow because these accessory muscles require more energy but still only marginally generate sufficient inspiratory flow. Recovery often involves stabilizing the chest while leaning forward with hands on the knees or sitting at a table with elbows supported. And, of course, lying flat in bed is next to impossible as several pillows will be needed to elevate the chest.

What causes emphysema? Although smoking is the first thing that comes to mind there's more to it than that. Let's look at just a little more physiology: The human body contains a large amount of elastic fibers. Little stretchy tissues that, when stretched a bit, are able to recoil and return to their original shape. The two most prevalent elastic fibers are **elastin** and **collagen**. They provide the structure for skin as well as all internal organs and blood vessels. Since breathing requires the lungs to expand and recoil with each breath the lungs contain a large amount of these elastic fibers. They have to, otherwise exhalation would require actively pushing out each breath. Although these elastic fibers last a long time, their elasticity gradually diminishes with aging. Around age 30 the production of collagen begins to decrease and the results begin to be noticeable throughout the body. Skin, joints and lungs just don't have the elasticity they once had. After all, wrinkle cream is marketed to the elderly, not to teenagers. Although aging *does not* result in emphysema, as aging progresses, the predicted lung function gradually decreases. And although each of us varies slightly in this process, most people's activity levels seem to diminish in proportion to aging. Unfortunately, smoking is known to accelerate the aging process. It's an attention getter when a 45-year-old smoker is told that their lung function is normal for an 80-year-old. A common misconception among smokers is that when breathing becomes a problem they'll just quit, go to the gym, work out and get their lungs back in shape. Unfortunately, it doesn't work that way.

Not all smokers will develop emphysema. In fact, only about 30% develop significant emphysema during their lifetime to the extent that normal activities of daily living will be severely disrupted. Sometimes one has little control over environmental pollutants, but smoking, as well as secondhand smoke, is something that can and should be avoided. Even though the lungs are inside the body, their health is directly related to what's outside, i.e., the air breathed.

Although smoking is a major contributor, what about those who have never smoked and have severe emphysema—does it run in families? Absolutely. An inherited deficiency called **alpha-1 antitrypsin (AAT)** is a known cause of emphysema, and although it is not common, a family history of lung disease or a personal history of frequent URIs should alert one to discuss this with the doctor. Although AAT is a complex problem, let's try to simplify it: Whenever one catches a URI an inflammatory response will result. The body responds by releasing enzymes which help to destroy the germ membranes. Unfortunately, they also destroy some of those elastic fibers in the lungs. The liver produces AAT to minimize the damage to these elastic fibers and help protect the lungs. If the liver is unable to produce the AAT in sufficient quantity or shape, more elastic fibers will be lost every time a URI occurs. In other words, the lungs will be aging much faster even without additional risks. Although nothing will reverse the damage already done, testing for AAT is available. Results may guide the physicians to a treatment plan and minimize further lung damage. Perhaps more importantly, knowing that a genetic link to lung disease is present may help other family members to minimize lung damage before it occurs. Simple blood tests are available to check for the presence of this gene. Free tests may be available through the national AAT association. Just call them.

Although chronic bronchitis and emphysema, the two entities of COPD, differ in nature, they are similar in outcome—breathing is a major problem. But what about asthma? Breathing is also a problem with asthma, and small children who have never smoked can have asthma. Is asthma yet another form of COPD, or is it like allergies, and what's the difference?

Asthma: Although asthma is not included in the classification of COPD, for many, the symptoms are a frequent struggle which seem to be chronic in nature. Is it possible to have asthma and COPD at the same time? Unfortunately, the answer is yes. Referred to as **asthma-COPD overlap syndrome (ACOS)**. Although the symptoms are similar, determining the difference can be difficult. The primary difference with asthma is that breathing can progress from normal to bad but return back to normal when the symptoms are controlled. COPD, on the other hand, usually fluctuates between "bad" and "worse." Asthma is the more common name for what is more accurately described as **hyperactive airway disease**. This simply means that the immune system's protection

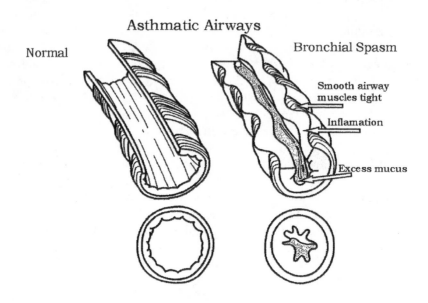

Asthmatic airways.

of the airways is just too sensitive and it overreacts. Nevertheless, whatever it's called, there are two distinct problems with asthma.

The first problem is called a **bronchial spasm**, which occurs when the smooth muscles which support the smaller bronchial tubes overreact and tighten. Let's use an extreme example to illustrate: While washing a load of clothes and adding bleach, one accidently gets a good whiff of the caustic bleach fumes. First the eyes, nose and trachea would immediately respond by flooding those areas with mucus. The smaller bronchial tubes will immediately spasm and constrict to minimize the damage downstream. And this is exactly how they're designed to work, but unfortunately, breathing is still something that has to continue. A bronchial spasm can occur very rapidly, and often results in the characteristic **wheeze**. The wheeze is nothing more than air trying to get through a diameter that is too small. While blowing air out of the mouth, and gradually constricting the lips, a whistle will be heard. Now multiply this whistle by thousands of small tubes restricting the flow, the single whistle becomes a wheeze. It was once thought that everything that wheezed was asthma but that couldn't be farther from the truth. For example, a child who swallows a coin will have a partially obstructed airflow and could have a wheeze without an actual bronchial spasm.

Excessive mucus, which is partially blocking the bronchial tubes, may also cause a wheeze. A wheeze doesn't necessarily diagnose asthma but it does indicate that something is wrong. There is, however, a big difference between wheezing while inhaling as opposed to wheezing while exhaling. During inhalation, the increasing air pressure helps to splint the airways open and wheezing is less likely. The opposite happens during exhalation, where the airways are more likely to be more forcibly constricted. This is especially noticeable during forceful exhalation. Therefore, wheezing upon exhalation is one thing but wheezing during inhalation is a lot more serious.

One additional note here concerning abnormal-sounding breathing; **strider**. This is a harsh vibrating, barking sound noticed in the larynx (voice box) area rather than the lungs (chest). It is not normally associated with symptoms of asthma or COPD but rather suggests a partial obstruction in the area of the vocal cords. In children, this area is proportionally smaller as compared to an adult so even a minor inflammation could result in these abnormal sounds, more often called **croup**. Since a partial obstruction of the airway occurs, it needs to be evaluated by a physician.

The second problem is inflammation of the walls of the bronchial tubes. The inflammation is a protective response by the immune system to thicken the walls of the bronchial tubes. Thicker walls are more stable than thinner walls. Unfortunately, the walls of the bronchial tubes are expanded inward, further decreasing the diameter and restricting airflow. As often happens during an acute asthma attack, inflammation and increased mucus production along with bronchial spasms significantly limit the ability to breathe. And since breathing is absolutely essential for life, it's no wonder that asthma-related problems remain one of the leading causes of death in the world. It's been estimated that 1 in 12 people has an asthmatic condition, and the number is continuously increasing. And scientists aren't really sure why this is, but they all agree that asthma is much more complex than just allergies. There are several subsets of asthma and it is not uncommon for patients to exhibit a little of each.

Extrinsic asthma is essentially triggered by substances external to the body that the immune system has determined may be harmful. When exposed to such substances, the body aggressively responds with an inflammatory response to the airways. Evidence suggests that an inherited tendency is likely, since these traits often run in families, including a hypersensitivity to viruses and bacteria. In other words, with extrinsic asthma it's easy to catch whatever is going around. A thorough examination including testing and review of one's medical history is necessary to identify specific allergens vs. environmental irritants. Normally, the immune system is not fully developed until humans reach puberty, so it's not surprising that extrinsic sources are most often responsible for asthma in children. Of course, avoiding these exposures will minimize the response. However, some studies, such as the **hygiene hypothesis theory**, suggest that letting children develop in an environment that is too clean deprives the immune system from developing properly. Whether or not letting the kids play in dirt is a "scientific" approach, it's generally frowned upon by most medical authorities. However, letting kids be kids, experiencing their surroundings and allowing their immune systems to develop, seems to be a more reasonable alternative. Those who have lived their adult lives in a certain area and later move to a totally different climate may spend the first few months with allergy-like symptoms. The likely cause is the different grasses and pollens that their immune systems have never encountered. The immune system doesn't recognize this new allergen and responds appropriately. After a few months the immune system adapts to the newer environment and symptoms usually subside.

Intrinsic asthma, unlike extrinsic asthma, are non-seasonable, non-allergenic circumstances which usually occur later in life and tend to be chronic in nature. Although the usual triggers, as mentioned earlier, may continue to be a factor, emotional responses such as laughing, crying or fright may bring about bronchial spasms. Exercise-induced asthma, where symptoms are noticed during or after a physical workout, are also classified here. Hormonal changes, as one goes through life, also seem to play a role as a possible contributing factor. This could help explain why some have symptoms at an early age yet "grow out of it" later in life, while for others, it's the other way around.

Eosinophilic asthma is also known as **atopic asthma**. This is not a common form of asthma but is one that usually doesn't respond well to traditional therapies. It is more often diagnosed in middle-aged adults with persistent asthmatic symptoms. Eosinophils are a normal component of the immune system whose numbers are increased during specific infections and promote inflammation. As the infection diminishes, the number of eosinophils returns to normal. However, some patients retain an abnormally high eosinophils count, resulting in persistent inflammation. Therapy is intended to diminish the number of circulating eosinophils.

Whatever the cause, all experts agree that asthma is a complex problem and usually involves multiple triggers which results in symptoms. Although the body's response to the triggers may be appropriate, that doesn't lessen the distressful symptoms of shortness of breath. However, with asthma, the immune system has misjudged some substances to be more harmful that they actually are. Trace amounts of automobile exhaust, diesel fumes, perfume, cigarette smoke, food ingredients and cold air just to name a few. To complicate the situation even more, symptoms *sometimes occur only* when combinations of these triggers occur together. A physician specializing in allergy testing may be of help. Additionally, many patients have helped narrow the search by playing the role of detective in the search for possible triggers. And best yet, it doesn't cost anything to make a daily journal of those you can identify.

Keep this journal for two weeks and use a different piece of paper each day. At the end of two weeks, sit down and sort the papers into three piles based on question #1. Now go through each of the three piles and look to see what the answers in each pile have in common. It just may be possible to identify combinations that could be avoided and reduce the possibility of an attack. Other times avoidance may not be possible, but it doesn't cost anything to try.

1. How was my breathing today:
    (a) Normal, no problems; didn't really have to think about it too much today
    (b) Some problems but I wasn't limited in what I wanted to do by my breathing
    (c) Had a lot of problems today and had to stop often because of my breathing.
2. What was the weather like today:
    (a) Nice, no rain, sun shining, not too windy
    (b) Cloudy, rain/snow, hotter or colder than normal, windy
        (c) I was indoors most of the day
        (d) I was outdoors often today
3. How was my sleep last night:
    (a) Normal amount, felt rested
    (b) Restless night, didn't feel rested
4. Stress levels today:
    (a) Easy going day, enjoyed myself
    (b) Obstacles just seem to get in my way today, but I overcame them easily
    (c) Lots of stress at work/home today, nothing went right
5. What did I have to eat and drink today:
    (a) Breakfast/snack:
    (b) Lunch/snack:
    (c) Supper/snack:
6. What was your best Peak Flow Measurements today: *(discussed in chapter 4)*
7. What physical activities or exercise did I do today:
8. Anything else that happened today that was different:

Asthmatic assessment worksheet.

Asthma-COPD Overlap Syndrome (ACOS): When you're unable to breathe, the last thing you're going to worry about is if it's asthma or COPD. But to help better manage these problems, a pulmonologist will need to evaluate your symptoms, history, lab and a breathing test to determine a proper plan of care. Although symptoms of shortness of breath, coughing and wheezing are common to both asthma and COPD, symptoms of chest tightness are more often seen in asthma as opposed to COPD. Although there are numerous exceptions, a history of smoking and other hazardous environmental factors is more common with COPD than asthma.

The most definitive information will come from the **pulmonary function test (PFT)**. Breathing into a **spirometer** that measures the volume and speed of airflow into and out of the lungs will help with diagnosis of the problem. Both asthma and COPD will slow the flow of air from the lungs on a forced exhalation. However, inhalation of a medicine to relax the smooth muscles of the bronchial tubes (rescue medicine) often significantly improves the results in asthmatics but is less effective with COPD. The amount of air residing in the lungs during normal breathing (**residual volume**) will be higher in COPD but may in fact be normal with asthmatics. Although there are many similarities and very often the course of treatment is similar, having an accurate diagnosis will help the doctor to develop a better plan of care.

Once the diagnosis has been made, the plan of care developed will likely include a variety of medications. Various pharmaceutical strategies may be needed, since there may be a number of reasons why breathing is a problem. And of course, sometimes the breathing problems may have nothing to do with the lungs. That's why it is important to see a pulmonary specialist who is trained and experienced to make a proper diagnosis. Without a proper diagnosis, appropriate treatment will be a process of trial and error. Taking a medication that doesn't address those problematic areas not only will be of limited value but could be dangerous and expensive as well. Let's take a look in the next chapter at the different classes of medication available and the various devices used to deliver them.

Additional Reading

Melinda Ratini, DO, MSN, 29 October 2020, "Asthma vs. COPD: What's the Difference?" www.webMD.com.
"Emphysema," 13 February 2020, www.drugs.com.
Laura J. Martin, MD, MPH, 17 November 2019, "Alpha-1 Antitrypsin (ATT) Deficiency," www.webMD.com.

3

Isn't There a Pill for That?

We are fortunate enough to have lived in the era of modern medicine. When we get sick, the doctor always has had something to quickly make us better. We now live in an "instant" world and just don't have the time to wait around and get better. Unfortunately, chronic lung disease can't necessarily be managed at that speed. There just isn't a magic pill that will instantly undo a problem that's taken years to develop. Rather than seeking a cure, a more realistic goal should be to manage and lessen the complications of the disease. Part of the management will be an assortment of medications, and a question often asked is which medicine is the best. The answer may sound flippant, but the truth is the best medicine is the one that works for you. As discussed previously, there may be multiple reasons why breathing is a problem, some of which have nothing to do with the lungs. That's where the doctor comes in. And having a better idea of what's causing the problem is fundamental to charting the proper course of management. A doctor who specializes in breathing problems is a **pulmonologist**. These physicians have completed extensive training in diagnosing particular breathing problems so the proper course of therapy can be started.

It only makes sense that when the lungs are involved, inhaling medicine directly into those airways will be an effective therapy. In fact, inhalation has been used for centuries, even predating ancient Egypt. Various plants and spices were burned and the smoke residue was inhaled. In more recent years, hand-pumped atomizers of the type used to dispense perfume have also been used for medicinal purposes. Of course, the size of the particle and precise dosages were highly variable. Before looking at the various classes of medication that may be inhaled, let's take a look at several of the most common devices used to deliver inhaled medicines.

In the 1940s mechanical compressors were used to aerosolize liquids. Solutions were drawn through a small tube and then met a high-pressure jet of compressed gas. The liquid was then blown against a partition, which further reduced the size of the aerosol. These were referred to as pneumatic jet nebulizers; today, they are often referred to as pneumatic **small volume nebulizers (SVNs)**. Although effective, the compressors were bulky and not well suited for use away from home. Today there are a variety of jet nebulizer styles available. Additionally, ultrasound nebulizers as well as those that use a high-frequency vibrating mesh are also used to nebulize solutions. Many of these are battery operated, allowing them to be portable.

In the early 1950s a self-contained device for dispensing aerosolized medication became available. Rather than using a bulky compressor, chemicals were added which produced the necessary pressure to jet the solution into a breathable aerosol. The pressurized aerosol canister using a chemical propellant is commonly referred to as a **metered dose inhaler (MDI)**. This device delivers a measured (metered) short burst of aerosolized medicine with each activation. Unfortunately, the propellant used was contributing to the depletion of the earth's ozone layer. After December 31, 2008, the propellant was changed from chlorofluorocarbons (CFC) to hydrofluoroalkane (HFA), which is less harmful to the ozone layer. Several years prior to this, pharmaceutical companies realized that changes were coming and developed a third option that doesn't require propellants.

A **dry powdered inhaler (DPI)** uses the patient's own inspiratory force to elevate the dose into the inspiratory flow and ultimately into the lungs. External compressors and propellants are not required. Although this method had been used as far back as the mid–1800s, modern devices are easier to use and allow for more precise dosing.

A newer device, the Respimat **Soft Mist Inhaler (SMI)**, offers the advantage of a portable metered dose of medication without the use of chemical propellants. The slower and smoother aerosol is less likely to provoke coughing. This inhaler's ease of use has reduced many of the coordination problems that many patients had between activation and inhalation.

Although each of these devices has its own advantages and disadvantages, it's the action of the medicine, not the device, that produces the desired results. However, using the device correctly and appropriately is of equal importance. Because of this, let's first of all explore the various classes of medicines that the doctor might prescribe. In the next chapter we'll discuss the proper use and pros/cons of each device more thoroughly.

Shortness of breath may have different origins, and therefore different strategies may be needed to ease the symptoms. Prescribed medicines target specific problematic areas. That's why it's important to understand how they are supposed to help in order to report back to the doctor if they are working as planned.

Very often the only information provided to patients is "Here, this will make breathing easier." However, a better understanding of how these medicines bring about relief as well as being aware of potential complications will be helpful in managing one's care. In order to understand this a little better, we'll first have to look at a little more physiology. And although this subject can get quite complicated, let's try to keep it simple.

Think of medicines like a key and a lock. The key is an **agonist**, which is a chemical or hormonal molecule that binds to a **receptor** (the lock). That specific agonist will only fit that specific receptor lock. When the agonist binds to its corresponding receptor, specific nerves will be stimulated to release chemical messengers to cause a reaction. Throughout the body there are billions of receptors of various shapes and sizes. Some reside on the cellular membrane while others are within the cell itself. When appropriately stimulated, some will result in a fast and strong reaction, while others offer only a partial but more sustained response. Still others may bind to the receptor but not activate a response, thereby blocking the pathway. Many drugs used today have an effect similar to naturally occurring body agonists.

So what causes those unwanted side effects? It so happens that getting the correct key to the appropriate lock is actually a little complex. It's kind of like a billiards cue ball being shot into a full rack. Multiple receptors may need to be activated in order to ultimately result in the desired effect. The unwanted side effects may be the result of hypersensitivity or an appropriate but exaggerated response such as a fast heart rate. An allergic reaction, however, is a response by the immune system to a substance that is interpreted as harmful. When this happens, various substances such as histamine are released to cause an inflammatory response. These reactions may range from a mild rash to severe facial and tongue swelling (anaphylaxis) that could be life-threatening. That's why it is important to understand what the doctor is prescribing and report unusual unwanted side effects.

When it comes to breathing problems, bronchodilators are the most commonly prescribed medication. "Broncho" refers to the bronchial tubes and "dilate" means to increase the diameter, making it easier to breathe. Bronchodilators are of a class called **sympathomimetic drugs**. These medications target the responses the **autonomic nervous system** makes when stimulated. The autonomic nervous system handles all those important things we don't have time to think about. Like how fast the heart should beat or when to take the next breath. The sympathetic response is often referred to as the **fight-or-flight** response when adrenaline is released and provides a jolt of energy. This sympathetic response is designed to help us survive an emergency by setting up a cascade of responses that will improve the chance of survival during life-threatening events.

For example, let's say while you are walking down the street one evening, a big dog jumps out of the bushes and starts snarling. Without even thinking about it, the brain immediately initiates a response to improve the chance of survival. A heart rate of 60 won't be sufficient, so it instantly ramps up by beating faster and more forcefully. The blood vessels in the skin will begin to constrict, shifting more blood to the muscles where more power is needed. Since fight or flight will also require a greater exchange of air, the smooth muscles of the bronchial tubes will relax, opening up the airways (dilatation) and making breathing easier. Because survival may depend on an immediate response, these systems are tied to receptors known as **adrenergic receptors**. When activated, they immediately cause each of the systems to respond appropriately. This is why some of those side effects may make things a little jumpy.

The name for the class of bronchodilator medicines prescribed to open the airways, sympathomimetics, refers to how they they mimic (or "make like") the sympathetic response. The receptors that are involved here are the **alpha** and **beta adrenergic receptors**, which when stimulated activate the whole cascade of responses. Fortunately, over the years, the various subsets of receptors have been better identified. As a result, drugs have been developed to target only these receptors, thereby limiting many of the undesirable side effects of the medications. It's the **beta-two (B_2) receptors** that are more specific for bronchodilation and to a lesser extent the cardiovascular system.

Bronchodilators are offered in two classes: Those that are fast acting but have a limited duration (rescue medicines) and those that have a slower onset but longer duration. Just which strategy will work best for any patient will likely be a "trial" of starting with minimal medicines and progressing as needed. For some, using fast-acting bronchodilators may be sufficient for occasional needs. Others may need to use them on a regular scheduled basis and supplement with extra doses as needed. Still others do well with only the slower onset but longer duration bronchodilators, while others need a combination of both. All of these medications have potent side effects, and the ultimate dose will be the minimal amount that will provide a reasonable amount of relief without overdoing it. The doctor will then be able to refine the plan of care. Although the list of available medications is constantly changing, let's look at some of the more commonly used pulmonary medicines and the method used to dispense them.

Commonly Prescribed Short-Acting B_2 Adrenergic Agonists

Short-acting bronchodilators are often referred to as **rescue meds**. These are most effective as an inhaled product that, when coming into direct contact with bronchial B_2 receptors, reacts quickly to elicit a response of bronchodilation. Although the next two classes (methylxanthenes and anticholinergics) are also B_2 agonists, their actions are slightly different and therefore they are listed separately.

Albuterol (salbutamol) via SVN and MDI
MaxAir (pirbuterol) via MDI
ProAir (albuterol sulfate) via MDI and DPI
Proventil (salbutamol) via SVN and MDI
Serevent (salmaterol) via MDI
Ventolin (salbutamol) via SVN and MDI
Xopenex (levalbuterol) via SVN and MDI

Commonly Prescribed Long-Acting Bronchodilators (LABDs)

LABDs differ from the rescue meds in that they are designed to be absorbed by the lung cell membranes. Then they are slowly released back outside the membranes and slowly react with the B_2 receptors. As a result, they are not designed as a rescue medication but rather for maintaining a prolonged bronchodilation. It is also highly recommended that they be used in conjunction with a corticosteroid (to be discussed below). In 2003, after-market research showed an increased number of unexplained deaths in asthmatic patients using LABDs. The FDA then issued a **black box warning** label to be affixed to the packaging of some of these products. This included a warning of possible adverse reactions and deaths in asthmatics using LABDs. The exact nature of these harmful reactions was never fully determined. It is believed that during acute bronchial spasms, LABD, rather than the rapid-acting B_2 agonist, was used as the primary therapy. Additionally, if significant inflammation were present, airway blockage could suddenly occur toward the end of the current LABD dosage. In 2016, additional studies showed that when LABD *and* corticosteroids were used together, and used appropriately, the rate of asthma deaths did not increase. The warning has since been removed from some of these products. This also underscores the importance of understanding each of the medications that are being taken, what they will and will not do. At any rate, before beginning use of a LABD therapy always discuss these concerns with the doctor.

> Arcapta Neohaler (indacaterol) via DPI
> Brovana (arformoterol) via MDI
> Foradil (formoterol) via MDI
> Performist (formoterol) via SVN
> Tudorza Pressair (aclidinium bromide) via DPI

Methylxanthenes: The active component of these drugs, **theophylline**, has been widely used since the early 1900s. Methylxanthenes are naturally occurring substances found in coffee and tea (caffeine) and cocoa beans (theobromine). Holistic articles often promote natural cures for asthma; unfortunately, that would take a lot of coffee and chocolate before the wheezing stopped. Although classified as a weak bronchodilator, methylxanthenes offer other advantages. The effects of sympathetic receptor stimulation (fight-or-flight) will ultimately dissipate due to the release of **phosphodiesterase** by the **parasympathetic** nervous system. The parasympathetic system is often called the **rest and digest** system and simply resets things back the way they were before the sympathetic receptors were stimulated. By inhibiting phosphodiesterase, the net result of methylxanthene dosage is a prolonged bronchodilator effect. Additionally, mild increased sensitivity to carbon dioxide production as well as diaphragmatic contractibility also stimulate breathing. In some patients the production of **leukotriene** may be decreased, which helps reduce inflammation. Although methylxanthenes are useful drugs, therapeutic dosing is variable and symptoms of nausea are not uncommon. Newer generations of longer-acting bronchodilators have reduced this drug's role.

Commonly prescribed methylxanthene preparations which are theophylline based and normally administered in a variety of forms, including IV, syrup or tablet form, are

> Aminophylline (theophyllin & ethylediamine) via IV, tablet, syrup
> Theo-Dur (theophyllin) via tablet, syrup
> Theoair (theophyllin) via tablet, syrup
> Uniphyl (theophyllin) via tablet, syrup

Anticholinergics: The drugs in this class are also bronchodilators but they work in a slightly different way by blocking acetycholine (AcH) and the parasympathetic impulses. They also decrease the production of saliva and mucus. They are often used together with sympathometics for a better result.

Commonly Prescribed Anticholinergics (# short acting, * long acting)

> \# Atrovent (ipratropium bromide) via SVN as well as MDI.
> \# Combivent (Albuterol & Atrovent) as DuoNeb via (SVN) or
>   Combivent via MDI, Respimat
> * Incruse Eilipta (umeclidinium) via DPI
> * Seebri Neohaler (glycopurrolate) via DPI
> * Stiolto (tiotbopium bromide & olodateral) via Respimat
> * Spiriva (tiotropium) via DPI, Respimat
> * Tudorza Pressair (aclidinium) via DPI
> * Yupelri Pro (revefenacin) via SVN

Corticosteroids are a class of drugs that decrease inflammation, which is one of the primary complications of airway disease. Steroids therefore play a crucial role in the management of asthma and COPD. Let's examine a little more physiology to see how they work. In all tissues throughout the body are a group of cells known as **mast cells**. They are part of the early immune system response and act as sentinels. When stimulated by injury, infection or irritation, they release various chemicals that cause inflammation. Let's take a look at something we've all encountered and perhaps it will make a little more sense: coming down with an upper respiratory infection (URI). Since the viruses that cause URIs are often airborne, symptoms are usually first noticed in the nose. The ever-on-guard immune system quickly identifies the culprit and causes the mast cells to release **histamine**. This sets up a cascade of events that do a couple of things. The cells surrounding this area open their cellular "windows" and flood the area with their fluid. This dilutes the germs and causes sneezing, effectively expelling some of the viruses. The area is now swollen with cellular fluid and slightly elevates the local temperature. This hastens to the scene more of our immune-fighting squad whose job is to eliminate anything that shouldn't be there. While this battle is going on, the unpleasant part is the constant sneezing and wiping of our irritated nose. However, there's a purpose behind this because the friction increases blood circulation to the area, which speeds things along. A hypersensitive reaction to inhaled irritants such as pollen follows a similar route: histamine along with other substances are released for the same reason. And what do we do about it? We take ***anti***histamines, of course. Although mother nature has a plan in place, we just want to hurry things along.

Corticosteroids are similar to a natural steroid called **cortisol** which is produced in glands around the kidneys. It's important to note that when taking a prescribed steroid, the body stops making cortisol but gradually returns to its normal production in a few days when the prescribed steroids are stopped. That's why it is very important to never stop a prescribed steroid "cold turkey" unless specifically ordered to by the doctor. Normally, they will gradually taper the steroid down over a few days to allow the body to resume production of cortisol. Corticosteroids are not the same as the steroids that some athletes have abused. Those are called **anabolic steroids** and are completely different from the corticosteroids. The anabolic steroids increase masculine characteristics and muscle building. Corticosteroids, however, decrease inflammation. As beneficial as these miracle drugs are, there are serious side effects which can be bothersome. Most common are increased blood sugar, fluid retention, bruising, anxiety and weight gain. More importantly, though, since the action of steroids is to reduce inflammation, which is the immune system's first response to fighting infections, the risk of infection is increased. Therefore, be extra cautious of any suspicious symptoms and promptly take care of any minor cuts and scrapes. In emergency situations where **prednisone** is often administered via IV, weaning patients a few days later with oral dosages can reduce undesirable side effects of the drug. And as troubling as these side effects may be, they often go away once steroids are no longer needed. Or as one physician summed it up: "I can treat temporary side effects, but if my patient stops breathing, I can't help a dead person." Fortunately, the side effects of inhaled corticosteroids used for maintenance are relatively few, with one notable exception: Following inhalation of corticosteroids, it is important to always rinse the mouth with water and swish and spit several times. A yeast infection called **thrush**, resulting in a severe sore throat, is a potential problem for some patients, but the risks are minimized with regular rinsing.

Commonly Prescribed Inhaled Corticosteroids

Aerobid (flunisolide) via MDI
Aerospan (flunisolide) via MDI
Alvesco (ciclesonide) via MDI
ArmonAir RespiClik (fluiticasone) via DPI

Arnuity Ellipta (fluticasone) via DPI
Asmanex (mometasone) via MDI
Azmacort (triamcinole) via MDI
Beclovent and QVAR (beclomethasone) via MDI
Flovent (fluticasone) via MDI
Pulmicort (budesodine) via MDI and SVN

Combination drugs containing a <u>corticosteroid</u> as well as a *long-acting bronchodilator*:

Advair (<u>fluticasone-propionate</u> & *salmeterol*) via MDI and DPI
Anoro Ellipta (<u>umeclidinium</u> & *vilanterol*) via DPI
BREO Ellipta (<u>fluticasone</u> & *vilanterol*) via DPI
Dulera (<u>mometasone</u> & *formoterol*) via MDI
Symbicort (<u>budesonide</u> & *formoterol fumarate dihydrate*) via MDI

Combination drugs containing an <u>anticholinergic</u> as well as a *long-acting bronchodilator*:

Bevespi Aerosphere (<u>glycopyrrolate</u> & *formoterol fomarate*) via MDI
Stiolto Respimat (*olodaterol* & <u>tiotropium bromide</u>) via MDI
Utibron Neohaler (*indacterol* & <u>glycopyrrolate</u>) via DPI

Combination drug containing an <u>anticholinergic,</u> a *long-acting bronchodilator*, and a corticosteroid:

Trelegy Ellipta (umeclidinium & *vilanterol* & <u>fluticasone</u>) via DPI

Leukotriene Blockers and Mast Cell Stabilizers

Mast cells contain more than just the histamines they release. They also contain **leukotrienes,** naturally occurring substances that promote inflammation. The action of leukotriene blockers is to prevent these inflammatory substances from being released. Some drugs in this class are designed to prevent the binding of leukotrienes to the receptor sites. It's like putting the plastic safety plug in the electrical socket to keep the kids from sticking something in there and getting shocked. Others prevent the formation of leukotrienes, while others kind of "double bag" the mast cells to keep the things in there and from causing problems.

Commonly Prescribed Leukotriene Blockers

Accolate (zafirlukast) via MDI and tablet (leukotriene blocker)
Intal (cromolyn sodium) via MDI (stabilizes mast cell)

Singulair (montelukast sodium) via DPI and as a tablet
(leukotriene blocker)
Tilade (nedocromilsodium) via MDI (stabilizes mast cell)
Zyflo (zileuton) via tablet (inhibits formation of leukotrienes)

Monoclonal Antibody Therapy (Anti–IgE Therapy)

Drugs in this class are **biologics**. They are sometimes used to treat **allergic asthma**, also known as **atopic asthma**, which is caused by inhaled antigens resulting in persistent symptoms that are not well controlled by conventional therapy. Prior to beginning therapy, specific blood tests will be done; also, a detailed history of response to conventional therapy as it relates to the persistence and severity of symptoms. Biologics are not steroids but rather work by inhibiting **immunoglobulin antibodies (IgE)**, which are involved with allergic responses. These biologics target naturally occurring white blood cells known as **eosinophils** which are a normal component of the immune system. Normally, when infections or antigens are detected, the body temporarily increases the production of eosinophils. This causes swelling, which is our immune system's first line of defense. Unfortunately, if the symptoms are uncontrolled for a prolonged period, the increased eosinophils can actually worsen the inflammation. **Eosinophilic asthma** is a term that describes these exacerbated (prolonged) asthma attacks. Therefore, when conventional therapy has been less than optimal, biologics may be added to current therapy. By reducing the amount of circulating eosinophils, the excessive inflammation may also be reduced. These biologics are administered by injection usually once a week for 2–4 weeks or as determined by the doctor. They are currently not recommended for patients under age six or for patients with COPD where allergic asthma is not a factor.

Currently Prescribed Biologics

Cinqair (reslizumab) via injection
Dupixent (dupilumab) via injection
Fasenra (benralizumab) via injection
Nucala (mepolizumab) via injection
Xolair (omalizumab) via injection

If you are not familiar with any of the medications that have been listed, don't be dismayed. New products are regularly being introduced, just as older ones are removed from production all the time. Does a product being new automatically mean it's better, or when one is no longer available does it mean that it is no longer useful? Not necessarily. Newer formulas drive the market and less profitable ones are often discontinued. Although manufacturers may argue otherwise, drugs in the same class generally reach the same receptors as others in the same class. Something to consider though, is that the longer one stays with the same formula, after a while, it may become less effective in achieving the same response. In this case, changing to a different drug in the same class, with a slightly different formula, could be more effective. As always, be sure to discuss the cost/benefit with the doctor *and* pharmacist.

When a patient is admitted to a hospital quite often the medicines that are provided are different than what the patient normally takes at home. Two things here: first, the home medicines are largely maintenance doses—to keep things from getting worse. If hospitalization is now required, then things got worse, so some, at least temporary, changes are probably necessary. Also, hospitals just can't stock every medicine in the world, so one may find that the hospital must substitute other drugs in the same class for one's previously prescribed home meds.

If the nurse brings in medicine that's unfamiliar, ask for clarification. They need to explain what it is, what it's for and any side effects to watch out for. If you have questions that they are unable to answer (unless that is, it's an emergency) ask them to call the doctor. An explanation of "because the doctor ordered it" is not sufficient.

Some patients prefer to bring their home medicines to the hospital for use. If the attending doctor is in agreement, that's fine. The hospital pharmacist will still need to review all the home meds to assess compatibility with any new drugs being administered. However, problems arise when home meds are stashed in a bedside table and continue to be taken according to the home schedule. If you are receiving scheduled breathing treatments several times a day while (unknown to the nurses) the home rescue inhaler is also being used, the doctor will be overestimating your response. The nurses need to know what is being taken and when. Duplications of medicines will likely present problems. I have often seen patients with multiple rescue inhalers, usually all in the same class but marketed under different names. Always check with the doctor *and* pharmacist.

Occasionally doctors will prescribe medicines for purposes other than what they were designed and marketed for. This falls under the category of **off-label** prescriptions. As mentioned earlier, the agonist (key) may have to unlock additional receptors (locks) which stimulate and/

or block additional reactions. If the results are favorable, that medicine could be prescribed for that reason even though it was tested and approved for a non-related condition. Once again, it is important to know your medications and openly communicate with the doctor and pharmacist.

Herbal and Integrative Remedies

Combinations of traditional pharmacological therapies, as mentioned above, as well as non-traditional strategies are favored by many; however, *always* thoroughly discuss any and all additives to the treatment plan with the doctor. Many over-the-counter supplements may interfere with the doctor's care plan.

Vitamin C and E (antioxidants): Free radicals are toxins that are byproducts of **metabolism** that result in "oxidative stress," which interferes with vital functions of the cell. Air pollution, smoking and fried foods are known to increase the production of free radicals. Vitamins that our body uses to naturally counteract this oxidative stress are called **antioxidants**, which help protect against cellular damage. Many fruits and vegetables contain high levels of antioxidants. Be sure to eat enough fruits and vegetables.

Omega-3 fatty acids: Studies have not demonstrated an improvement in lung function for those consuming more omega-3s; however, a diet higher in omega-3s may help control other chronic problems such as elevated cholesterol and heart disease that complicate good health and further exaggerate preexisting breathing problems.

Cough preparations: Chronic coughing is often a common symptom of pulmonary disease. Various over-the-counter products are available to minimize this distressful symptom. Always use caution when selecting a particular formula because not all cough medicines work the same. **Antitussive** cough products block (suppress) the cough reflex, and *dextromethorpham* is a common ingredient. This may be helpful if pulmonary secretions are not excessive (dry cough). **Expectorant** cough products tend to thin the pulmonary secretions, allowing them to be coughed up (expectorated) easier, and a common ingredient is *guaifenesin*. The important point here is that *not all coughs are the same*. If secretions are excessive and a cough suppressant is used, the secretions will stay in the airways and could block the flow of air. Other times, the cough may be the result of something other than pulmonary secretions, such as a side effect of other medicine. If there are any questions be sure and talk with the pharmacist.

Allergy testing and immunotherapy: Hypersensitivity to common environmental allergens can compound symptoms. If allergies are suspected, a doctor who specializes in allergy medicine can test for abnormal response to a variety of commonly found substances. If testing positive to any given substance, small doses of that substance may be administered over a period of time so your immune system has a chance to become adapted to it and therefore reduce inflammatory responses.

Meditation, tai-chi and yoga: Stress reduction is fundamental to managing any chronic condition, and shortness of breath certainly qualifies here. All these disciplines emphasize control of breathing, balance, movement and posture in order to manage stress.

Acupuncture, acupressure and chiropractic biophysics: These disciplines use the "road map" of our nervous system to alter stimulation to specific root nerves that may be either overstimulating or blocking systems, resulting in unwanted effects.

Lifestyle modifications: Topics that will be explored in the next few chapters, unfortunately are often overlooked when all that is wanted is a quick fix: Quitting smoking, adequate hydration, diet modification as necessary, developing a proper exercise program, keeping all immunization shots up to date, frequent handwashing, taking appropriate precautions in environmentally suspect environments as well as crowded spaces during cold and flu season and using all prescribed medications appropriately are all important pieces of a successful care plan. If lifestyle modifications are needed but not made, any therapeutic strategies implemented by the doctor will always be less than optimal.

As mentioned earlier, taking medications is only half the battle because if they are not taken properly the full benefit may not be reached. In fact, sometimes misuse can make things worse. Additionally, the price of prescription medicines is often a major issue for many people these days. Even for those fortunate enough to have health insurance *and* able to afford the co-pays, these things aren't cheap. Over the last few years, hospitals have seen a dramatic increase in the number of patients coming to the emergency department who have run out of medicines and can't afford more. Recently, I knew of a young woman who came to the emergency department with a mild case of pneumonia, was treated and discharged with a prescription for the appropriate antibiotics. She returned two weeks later, CPR in progress, and didn't survive—the prescriptions forms were still in her pocket—she couldn't afford them. Cases like hers shouldn't happen but they do. Let's look at the next chapter for some additional suggestions about obtaining and using medicines properly and safely to obtain the maximum benefit.

Additional Reading

Dan Brennan, MD, 20 December 2019, "Bronchodilators (Rescue Inhalers): Short and Long Acting Types," www.webMD.com.

Alan Carter, PharmD, 29 June 2019, "What You Need to Know about Bronchodilators," www.medicalnewstoday.com.

Carol DerSarkissian, 5 August 2019, "Bulk Up Your Steroid Smarts," www.webMD.

4

How Do I Take
This Breathing Medicine?

Following the first portion of the pulmonary function study, the doctor had ordered a bronchodilator to be administered. The test would then be repeated to measure the response. The patient told me that he would rather use his own MDI but it never really helped. He put the inhaler between his lips and took four puffs in quick succession. "You see?" he said. "Didn't do a thing." I sat back and asked him, "Do you see that little orange cap on this end? Why don't you take it off and try it again and see what happens?" As simple as that sounds, I've seen this scenario repeated numerous times over the years. Most of us are used to taking medicine for one thing or the other. Normally all that's necessary is to chuck it down the hatch and let it do its magic. Unfortunately for my pulmonary function patient, all he was getting out of his inhaler was a wet spot in his pocket. After I instructed him on the proper use of his MDI, he was surprised at how much better he was able to breathe.

A major problem in the United States today is the increasing cost of pharmaceuticals. And way too many people are being priced out of the market. Even when expense isn't an issue, prescriptions don't do much good if not used correctly. All too often the instructions are too vague. The package insert that comes with the prescription probably results in more confusion than ever. However, understanding that information can be the difference between improved health or making things worse. I recently took care of a young woman who had a severe asthma attack. In one day, she used the entire contents of her recently purchased steroidal MDI (an expensive $250 one), and didn't get any relief. Given that it was pricier than her $15 rescue inhaler, she thought it would be better. She should have read the last chapter. Fundamentally, all medicine is good *if* used for the right circumstance and *if* administered at the right time *and* in the right manner. My pulmonary function patient used the right inhaler but not properly. The asthma patient used her inhaler properly but used it for the wrong circumstance. Neither one benefited from their efforts.

Medication used in the management of COPD and asthma comes in various forms: liquids to be swallowed and liquids to be inhaled; pills to be swallowed and pills containing a powder to be inhaled. And if that weren't enough there are devices such as small volume (jet) nebulizers (SVNs), soft (slow) mist inhalers (SMIs), metered dose inhalers (MDIs), and dry powdered inhalers (DPIs). Which one works best—and is technique important? Let's take a look at the most commonly used devices and how to use them for the best results.

Metered dose inhalers (MDIs) are small and portable, making them ideal for use when away from home. As noted, it's important to know the contents of the inhaler, since it's the medicine not the device that will help. MDIs contain a pressurized canister and a holder which, when the canister is depressed, produces a measured dose of medicine in an aerosol. From a full canister, the velocity is at least 45 mph, and at that speed, about 80% will impact the back of the throat, which is not the intended target area. As a result, the effects are minimal at best. The "blast" from the MDI is not sufficient to propel the medicine

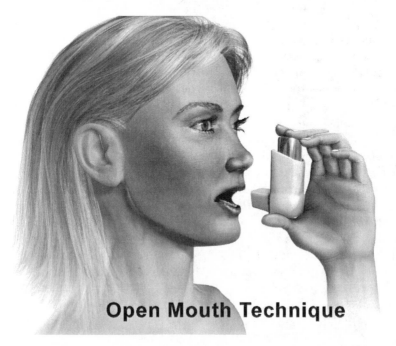

Open Mouth Technique

Metered dose inhaler open mouth (Bruce Blaus).

into the airway. The aerosol must be inhaled within a moving current of air. There are two ways to accomplish this: the open mouth technique or the use of a spacer. One requires an extra piece of equipment, the other only coordination. Unfortunately, many patients just "pop" it in their mouth and puff away because that's how they've seen others us it. Unfortunately, when used this way, not enough airflow is generated to carry sufficient aerosol into the lungs. In fact, only about 20% reaches any portion of the upper airways. And it's the lower airways where most of the bronchial spasms are occurring. Of course, if the MDI is placed between the lips but in front of the teeth, not even that much will reach the lungs. A better method is the open mouth technique, where the MDI is held about an inch away from the open mouth and discharged while slowly inhaling. The benefits are that now about 80% of the aerosol will be carried into the lungs. Not only will the results be better, not as many puffs will be needed for a favorable result. The net result is that the MDI will last about 60% longer, saving money. The only disadvantage to this technique is that some degree of coordination is required. Not that spraying the face will be harmful but it won't exactly help the breathing either.

A spacer device is a holding chamber that is attached to the MDI

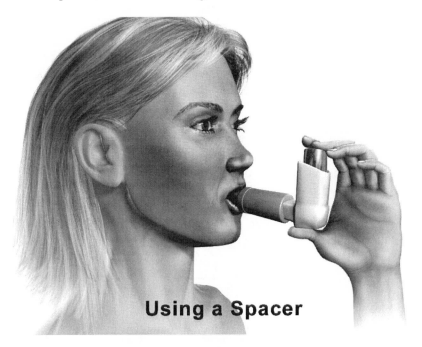

Using a Spacer

Metered dose inhaler spacer (adult) (Bruce Blaus).

orifice and will hold the aerosolized medicine. Additional room air will be entrained as the suspended aerosol is slowly inhaled. At the front of the spacer is a one-way valve to prevent the aerosol from being pushed out the mouthpiece. The valve, however, is easily opened during inspiratory flow. There are two drawbacks to the spacer. The first is that spacers are bulky and somewhat of an inconvenience to carry around, though unless the open mouth technique can be mastered, they'll be worth the effort. The other factor is cost. Spacers can vary in price from $10 to $50 and the added cost may be prohibitive. Fortunately, not all MDIs require their own type of spacer; so one holding chamber can be used with multiple inhalers. I've seen patients using an improvised spacer from the cardboard tube of an empty roll of toilet paper. Although this won't work as a holding chamber, it will direct the discharged aerosol into the mouth. And since airflow is able to be entrained at the rear of the tube, it seems to work fine. But if the few extra dollars are not prohibitive, a spacer is a good investment. There are now a few MDIs that have a spacer attached and others that produce a slow fine mist (Respimat) when activated rather than a rapid blast. As a result, the discharged aerosol is able to be carried with the inspiratory airflow and the results are greatly improved.

Whether using a spacer or the open mouth technique, an important sequence needs to be followed to ensure optimal results.

1. **Make sure the MDI isn't empty.** Shaking it a few times and listening for the "sloshing" sound is not a good indicator of the amount of medicine or pressure remaining. Most modern MDIs now have a volume counter as part of the mechanism, so look for it. If that particular MDI is used only for maintenance, it should be easy enough to mark the calendar when to buy a refill. If, however, the MDI is used as a rescue inhaler where use is irregular, be sure to check the counter frequently. In the event that the MDI doesn't have a counter, the volume left can be measured by doing a **float test** with a glass of water. Remove the cylinder from the holding chamber and approximate the volume of medicine remaining. If it sinks, it's nearly full. If it remains upright without sinking, about half full and if it lies on its side on the surface of the water, get a new one. Again, if it has a numerical counter as part of the holder, a float test is not needed so don't put it in water. In all cases, have a new one on hand before the one in use is empty.

2. **Shake the MDI about 10 times.** Shaking "excites" the propellant that causes the medicine to be aerosolized. If using a spacer, the MDI can stay attached as it is being shaken.

3. **The MDI** *may* **need to be purged.** As discussed in the previous chapter, after December 2008, the gas propellant was changed from CFC to HFA to comply with federal regulations. Unfortunately, the HFAs do not produce as strong of a propellant as the CFCs. If the MDI has not been used for a few days, it is possible for the activation chamber to become partially obstructed with dried medicine. If this is the case, the manufactures recommend that one puff be expended prior to the first activation. However, if the MDI has been used on a daily basis this shouldn't be necessary.

4. **Remove the protective cap.** Remember, if using a spacer device, it also may have a cap. They both need to be removed.

5. **Position your lungs to receive the aerosol.** Using the MDI while sitting or standing up straight, if possible, will allow for a deeper breath. A shallow inhalation may not carry sufficient medicine to the lower airways. Before starting, take a couple of slow deep breaths, then exhale fully. A full exhalation is important because the deeper the aerosol is inhaled into the lungs, the more lung surface area will be reached. If starting with the lungs half full of air, less surface area can be reached to absorb the aerosolized medicine.

6. **Place the device between the teeth and lips.** (a) *If using the spacer*, first position the lungs as in #5, then place the mouthpiece between the teeth and lips, depress the canister *once* to release the aerosol and slowly inhale deeply. Most spacers have a reed valve that will make a musical note if the inhalation is too fast. If hearing a harmonica type of sound while inhaling, slow down. A fast inhalation causes the air currents to become turbulent and jam up in the upper airways, limiting one's the ability to fully inhale. Visualize what would happen if you tried to fill an empty water bottle sitting under the faucet in the kitchen sink simply by turning the faucet on full blast. Water would splash out around the opening with little actually getting into the bottle. If, however, the flow were slower, the bottle would fill nicely. The same thing happens with currents of air; therefore, slow and steady does it.

   (b) *If using the open mouth technique*, Hold the MDI about an inch away from the open mouth. Position the lungs as in #5, then slowly begin the inhalation and (*without stopping*) activate the aerosol by depressing the canister *once* and continue inhaling until reaching a full breath. If the inhalation is stopped to depress the canister, most of the aerosol will end up in the mouth, not the lungs. The inhaled flow of air must be continuous to carry the aerosol along with it.

7. **Hold the breath.** At the end of that inhalation, the only aerosol medicine that is going to work is that which touches the lining of the airways. The airways are tubular and, as a result, much of the aerosol is still suspended in the middle of the airways, just waiting to be exhaled. By holding the inhaled breath for 5–10 seconds, this will allow some of that suspended aerosol to drop out of suspension and connect with the surface of the bronchial tube.

8. **Exhale with pursed lips.** At the end of that brief breath hold, exhale slowly, keeping a little bit of back pressure in the airways. By exhaling this way, even more suspended aerosol will have a chance to connect with the bronchial tubes. Pursed lip exhalation is kind of like a slow whistle. We'll discuss this much more in later chapters.

9. **Wait at least a minute before the next inhalation.** If requiring more than one puff, wait at least one minute between each puff. This will allow the inhaler to re-pressurize before the next dose. If the second puff is activated sooner, more of what is discharged will be propellant than the actual medicine.

MDI summary: Advantages are that the MDI is a portable device that can be used anywhere and is small enough to fit in a pocket or purse. A spacer or the open mouth technique should be used to provide optimal dosage; otherwise, additional equipment is not required. The disadvantages are primarily in the technique of use. If an MDI is not used in the manner described above, optimal dosing is less likely to be achieved and multiple activations will be required. Another disadvantage is cost. Medicare generally sets the standard, and unfortunately it's assumed that if one's breathing is that bad, one shouldn't be out and about but just sitting at home in the rocking chair using the (less expensive) nebulizer. Note, however, that some medications are only available as MDIs.

Small volume nebulizer: The most common nebulizer (jet) devices use a compressed source of air to siphon a small volume of liquid into position where the jet of air causes it to become aerosolized. The medications aerosolized are similar in dosages to the other devices. The primary difference is that the dose is delivered over the course of several minutes. Therefore, coordination is not as critical. A mouthpiece or aerosol face mask may be used, although a mouthpiece is the preferred interface. Unfortunately, between breaths, aerosolized medicine continues to be produced and exits the rear of the mouthpiece assembly and is therefore lost to the airways. To recover some of this lost aerosol, a short piece (about six inches) of large-bore tubing is attached opposite the mouthpiece. During the next inhalation, as room air is drawn in, the first portion will contain some of this "escaped" aerosolized medication. Normally, the ratio of inhalation to exhalation is 1:2 (exhalation twice as long), so it is expected that two-thirds of a normal nebulizer's production will be lost.

A device known as a **breath activated nebulizer (BAN)** produces an aerosol only upon inhalation and not during exhalation. Many hospital emergency centers are using a similar device in order to provide a comparable therapeutic dose of medicine in a shorter amount of time. The disadvantage for home use is the BAN nebulizer is much more expensive than the traditional nebulizer. Also, some compressors used at home don't generate sufficient compression to work with the BAN. The larger problem, however, is the temptation to use only one-third of the nebulizer solution, leaving it sitting in the nebulizer for later use. The danger here is cross contamination of the solution remaining in the nebulizer and increasing the chance of respiratory infections.

Small portable battery-powered nebulizers that use high-frequency mesh vibration to produce aerosol particles have become increasingly popular. Besides being portable, they are able to use the liquid medicine normally used in traditional nebulizers. For most insurance plans, the same medicine used in a nebulizer is much less expensive compared to that used as an MDI. Although manufactures will disagree, the particle size and ease of use are similar, so if cost is a factor, shop around.

But whichever nebulizer device is being used, breathing techniques similar to those described for use with the MDI should be employed, with *four important modifications.*

1. The nebulizer treatment will take about 5–15 minutes to complete, so don't rush it.
2. Obviously, breathing deeply with a breath hold following each inhalation will be exhausting. To reduce fatigue, breathe normally, but about every 10 to 15 seconds or so, take a deep breath and briefly hold it. This may initially be difficult, but after a few minutes, as the airways begin to open up, it should become easier.
3. Excessive coughing sometimes occurs during the first minute or so of the aerosol therapy. If this occurs, briefly take shallower breaths to allow the medicine to open the airways. The recommended breathing pattern should then be used.
4. The equipment needs to be regularly cleaned and maintained. The home care company who supplied the nebulizer system should have provided instructions for cleaning and maintenance. If not,

call them back. The compressor doesn't need much attention except changing the dust filter several times a year. The nebulizers come in a variety of styles with different cleaning methods. Some are disposable and replaced after a few days, others are reusable and need to be cleaned on a daily basis. Others are dishwasher safe but many are not. Some dealers offer (out-of-pocket) expensive solutions. In lieu of the solutions, hand-washing the nebulizer with mild soap and warm water, then immersing it in a solution of white vinegar in a 1:4 dilution with distilled water for 20 minutes, is often recommended. Then thoroughly rinse the nebulizer and cover with a towel to air dry overnight. Always make sure a clean nebulizer is ready to go while one is being cleaned. It's important to check with the home care company as to recommendations—because *to not clean the nebulizer is not an option.*

Respimat Soft Mist Inhaler (SMI): The more recent SMI technology offers several advantages over other modalities. The medication is delivered in a soft mist that is not likely to provoke coughing. All necessary components are included and neither environmentally detrimental propellants nor an external compressor are required. Although a spacer device is not needed, one can be used in special circumstances. Coordination of the delivery and inhalation is still important but not as critical as with the MDI or DPI. The liquid medication is pre-loaded, and following initial assembly the device is easy to use.

1. **No more guessing if you have enough.** A dosage indicator on the cartridge tracks the available doses remaining. It is not necessary to shake the device, as propellants are not used.
2. **Initial use purging is needed.** Prior to the initial use, several actuations will be necessary to position the medication for use. Sufficient solution is already available to account for this initial purging. Follow the directions to ensure that a fine mist is observed. If the device is not used for a few days, purging may again be necessary. However, if using the SMI on a daily basis this shouldn't be necessary.
3. **Positioning the lungs.** For the same reasons as described with MDIs, sit or stand up straight and take several deep breaths and then exhale fully.
4. **Place the mouthpiece between the teeth and lips** with the opening pointing toward the back of the throat.
5. **Slowly begin inhalation**, then press the dose release button while continuing to inhale.

6. **Hold the breath 5–10 seconds** for the same reasons as described with MDIs.
7. **Exhale through pursed lips** for the same reasons as described with MDIs.
8. **Follow the prescribed instructions for dosage depending on the medication used.**

SMI summary: Advantages are that all equipment needed is supplied with the medication. They are small devices, allowing for portability. Once the final dose has been administered, a locking device will automatically engage and a new cartridge and inhaler will be required.

Disadvantages are that limited medications are offered in the SMI format.

Dry powdered inhalers (DPIs): With these devices designed as an alternative to aerosol-based therapies, neither environmentally detrimental propellants nor an external compressor are required. The medication may be loaded into the inhaler in the form of a pill, while in other devices the medication is self-contained in the inhaler. Moving the mouthpiece into position actuates the dose available for inhalation. There is no need to purge the device prior to use. The success of the DPI therapy depends on a forceful inhalation generating sufficient flow to break up the powder into smaller portions so it can be carried into the airways. The technique for successful application is similar to that used with MDIs, with one exceptions (#3 below):

1. **No more guessing if you have enough.** DPIs that require loading of the powder in a pill form are pretty easy to figure out. Other devices, in which the medication is preloaded, have a counter that changes each time another dose is loaded. Unlike with an MDI, neither a spacer device nor the open mouth technique is needed.
2. **Positioning the lungs.** For the same reasons as described with MDIs. Sit or stand up straight and take several deep breaths and then exhale fully.
3. **Inhale sharply.** Place the mouthpiece between the teeth and lips then *a quick inhalation is necessary* to "pick up" the powder to be carried into the lungs. This is because the powder has more density and therefore heavier aerosolized particles requiring quick, forceful inhalation.
4. **Hold the breath 5–10 seconds.** For the same reasons as described with MDIs.
5. **Exhale through pursed lips.** For the same reasons as described with MDIs.
6. **Once is enough.** Currently most DPIs are used as maintenance

medicines and not as rescue inhalers. Unless otherwise directed by the doctor, multiple doses will be unlikely, but always follow the doctor's instructions.

DPI summary: Advantages are that all equipment needed is supplied with the medication. DPIs are small devices and, in many cases, disposable once all of the doses have been completed. The disadvantages are that limited medications are offered in the DPI format. Also, substantial inspiratory flow must be generated to carry the powder into the lungs. This limits its use for the very young, elderly, uncooperative or unresponsive patient. Although not common, some very hyperactive airway (asthmatic) patients may actually develop a bronchospasm as a result of the inhaled powder.

As we've seen, there are several different devices that may be used to deliver medicine to the lungs. Each has advantages as well as disadvantages. And although all of them are designed to be inhaled directly into the airways, each requires use of specific techniques that must be followed to be successful. In other words, to get optimal results, one must

1. Use the appropriate medicine.
2. Use it for the appropriate circumstance.
3. Use the appropriate delivery device in an optimal manner.
4. Use it in a timely manner.

Unfortunately, *timely manner* is an aspect that is not well covered in the instructions. Rescue medicines are often prescribed for use as needed, which usually is interpreted as "when short of breath," and as a result, they are habitually over- or underused. Using such meds too often when not they aren't needed may eventually lessen one's sensitivity to them plus elicit uncomfortable and potentially dangerous side effects. Conversely, waiting until a mild distress becomes an emergency is equally dangerous. That's why a thorough understanding of these first several chapters is important. The following chapters will assist you in making appropriate decisions as to what else you can do besides just cranking away on the inhaler.

How to use maintenance medications is pretty obvious when one is applying the "timely" aspect. Just following the doctor's recommendations should be sufficient, although, even at that there may be some fine-tuning that could optimize those results. But ease of breathing can fluctuate from day to day. What about those medications that are used on as-needed basis?

Let's start with the rescue medications. There are several scenarios that come into play here, so it's important to understand which direction one should follow. For patients with excessive pulmonary secretions, regular use of a bronchodilator may be helpful. Typically, early morning when coughing can be anticipated can be very tiring and stressful. Dilating the airways 15–20 minutes before attempting to expectorate is helpful. Allowing more air to get behind the secretions will facilitate a better result with less effort. However, the airways of a typical asthma patient tend to remain open and stable until some trigger causes them to constrict, resulting in wheezing and shortness of breath. In this case, the use of the rescue medicine would be appropriate on an as-needed basis only unless excessive secretions are involved, as noted above.

For patients where asthma is the primary problem, wouldn't it be helpful to know in advance if an asthma attack was in the early stages? A simple device can provide the information to measure the stability of the airways. The results can help predict the likelihood of an asthma attack several days in advance. A **peak flow meter (PFM)** is just such a device. This simple device is easy to use, painless and only takes a few seconds to use. It's also the best measurement to evaluate the stability of the airway. Instructions are very simple: About the same time every day, take a deep breath and "blast" the exhalation through the peak flow meter. Wait a few minutes and try it two more times and keep track of the best value.

The surface area of the lungs is extremely large. This is important because daily there are

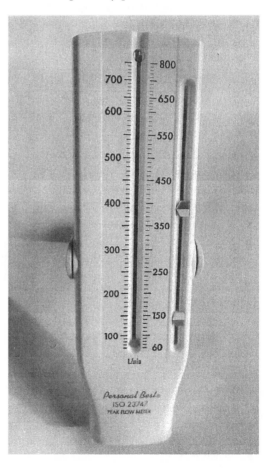

Peak flow meter Phillips Respironics Personal Best (Salicyna).

often small portions of the lungs (and airways) that aren't as open as they should be. Fortunately, there are plenty of other areas for the air to go. However, preceding an asthma attack, additional areas become partially blocked and the velocity of a forced exhalation is significantly reduced. Compare this to letting water run out of a hose while partially obstructing the opening with your thumb. The flow is partially obstructed and changes the spray pattern. And this is exactly what happens to airways when the bronchial tubes begin to spasm or inflammation is increasing. It's important to keep track of the daily measurements because a decrease in peak flow measurement from *your normal* is indicative of increased resistance to airflow.

Now, I emphasized "your normal," and this is very important. Included with the device will be a chart that will show **predicted peak flow** based on your sex, height and age. Forget that. You are *only* interested in changes from your normal values. Determining what that normal baseline value is usually takes a week or so of practice. The need to first establish a reliable, consistent and reproducible baseline is that important. It's important to establish this normal baseline while feeling well. If you're just recovering from an illness or asthma flare-up, wait until returning to a normal state of well-being before beginning. It's important to eliminate as many variables as possible such as changes in time of day, body position and use of meds.

Many find it convenient to put the PFM next to their toothbrush, since that's normally used about the same time each day. After a week or so, the values will start to fall around the same mark each day (+/- a little). Now that a normal baseline has been established, a distinct drop could indicate a potential problem. Even in the absence of other symptoms, a slightly reduced flow should alert one to pay a little more attention to breathing. More often than not, a reduced flow returns to normal the next day. If, however, on the next day the flow rate continues to drop, even though breathing is not difficult, consider using the rescue inhaler, just to stay ahead of things. Of course, if the measurements continue to decrease, call the doctor. This valuable tool provides a few days' head start in reducing or even preventing an impending asthma attack. Use it daily and track the results. Don't wait and lose the advantage of early treatment. Once again, the PFM is more useful for those whose breathing problems are confined to asthma (reactive airway disease) and less so for those with COPD.

When multiple inhaled medicines are prescribed, is there a sequence of which comes first? Actually, there is but the order could change from day to day and is due to the action of the medication itself. Remember that with any inhaled medication only that which touches the inside of the lower airways will be absorbed. Obviously, the deeper it's inhaled the more surface area will be reached, improving the results. If using a rapid-acting bronchodilator to open the airways as well as an inhaled steroid that gradually reduces inflammation, which should come first? I think I just gave it away, didn't I? That's why it's important to understand the action of each medicine so they can be used to their fullest advantage. Circumstances, however, change from time to time: severe distress and wheezing one day and not another; seasonal allergies at certain times of the year and not others. There may be times of the day where the side effects of some medicines interfere with one's activities. For those reasons it's important to have a thorough understanding of what the medications do and how to use them. Let's take a look at a few examples:

1. Rescue medications are typically reserved for sudden breathing problems. However, even when not in distress, many have found that using them first will optimize the use of other inhaled medicines. First dilating the airways and, about 20 minutes later, using other inhaled maintenance medication will allow for deeper penetration of maintenance inhalers.

2. Consider using the rescue medication prior to a planned exercise session. When one exercises, the rate and depth of breathing naturally increase and dry the airways. Optimize those airways first. Also consider using the rescue medication prior to attempting any task where increased exertion will be required, for example, lawn work or prolonged housecleaning.

3. What about when two medicines have similar actions; for example, a rapid-acting but short-duration bronchodilator and a slower-acting but longer-duration bronchodilator? Keep in mind that the short- and long-acting bronchial dilators are both competing for the same receptor sites. If both are needed, space them out by at least 30 minutes or so and circumstances should dictate the sequence: If experiencing a lot of trouble breathing, wheezing and shortness of breath, use the rapid-acting, short-duration (rescue) one first to quickly open the airways. Then later the longer-duration one could be used. When not in distress, use the slower-acting, longer-duration (LABD) one. The rapid-acting shorter-duration (rescue) could then be used later but *only* if needed. There very well may be times when the LABD is sufficient and the rapid-acting rescue medicine may not be needed. Therefore, the sequence may change depending on how one's breathing is at that particular time. One's need to alter this

sequence may very well change from day to day. That's why a better understanding of how and what those inhaled medicines do is likely to improve one's chances for optimal results.

4. A rapid-acting bronchodilator used late evening before bed can help to keep the airways open and allow easier breathing while sleeping. Unfortunately, the side effects could keep one jittery half the night, preventing sleep. Many patients find that the slower-acting but longer-duration bronchodilators, taken a few hours before bed, actually provide the relief needed without as many side effects.

5. Inhaled corticosteroids need to either be taken on a regular basis or not at all. If prescribed, they should be used daily as directed. Holding them in reserve and taking them only when feeling like you're "coming down with something," is not likely to help and in fact could actually make things worse. The action of corticosteroids is to hold back the immune system's response to infection or other irritation. When one is taking them for a few days, then stopping and starting again, the message to the immune system is confusing. Under these intermittent circumstances, the immune response will likely initiate an inflammatory response. The reasoning being that it's safer to have a positive result to a false alarm than the other way around.

6. Those affected with seasonal allergies already have a good working knowledge of when they are going to have problems. Therefore, medication may not be needed all year long. Arrange to begin use at least three weeks in advance of allergy season and continue for about a month past it.

In summary, prescribed inhaled medication may require a little more thought than just using it a few times a day as it says on the label. Talk with the doctor about these suggestions. All inhalers are not the same, just as the reasons for shortness of breath may not always be the same. Although the correct medication taken while using poor technique may ultimately be successful, proper technique will bring results more quickly and economically. As the cost of medicine continues to rise, cost-efficiency becomes more and more important. However, when one is out of breath, "quickly" is paramount.

By now you should have a better idea why doctors prescribe the specific classes of medicines they do for breathing troubles. And we have reviewed the commonly used devices used to deliver those medicines to where they are needed. However, beyond what the doctor or pharmacist can do, there are still a few more things that need consideration. What about affording them? Help may be available but where does one begin to look? Emergencies can happen at any time. Those coming to the rescue probably won't have any knowledge of your medical history. Can you rattle off your list of medications while gasping for air? What about a natural disaster, fire, flood, earthquake or hurricane—is there a plan in place? Situations beyond one's control always seem to pop up at the most inconvenient time. And as stress increases, things will be forgotten and breathing will continue to get worse. Let's look at the next chapter for suggestions on planning for those predicaments that can fall on our shoulders.

Additional Reading

"Peak Flow Meter," 9 April 2020, www.mayoclinic.org.
Ann Mulen, RN, CSN, 29 April 2018, "Devices for Inhaled Medications," www.national jewish.org.

5

What Else Do I Need
to Know About My Meds?

Understanding prescription medicines and taking them appropriately are fundamental to managing one's health. When you receive a new prescription from the pharmacy, instructions are provided on a lengthy piece of paper with print so small it can hardly be read. And then the pharmacy asks if you have any questions. What should one do? First of all, make sure to find a good pharmacist. These professionals are probably the most underutilized medical specialists today. When they ask if there are any questions, they really do mean it. The pharmacist on duty is the one trained to discuss exactly what is needed to be known about that new prescription. After all, when doctors have a question about various medicines, they call the pharmacist.

It's a good idea to make an appointment with a pharmacist to go over *all* your prescriptions and check for discrepancies. The time spent with them will be well worth the effort. Most pharmacies today use a computer to flag any drugs that could adversely react with one another. To be accurate, though, the pharmacy must have a complete list of all your medications. This includes any prescriptions from other pharmacies and all over-the-counter supplements. Although the prescribing doctor may very well have an appropriate strategy in mind for the use of various medications, what if there might be a better alternative? That's what a pharmacist is trained to do. They'll provide the needed information to be discussed with the doctor. A really good pharmacist will call the doctor themselves and say, "Hey, doc...?"

For convenience some prescriptions are automatically renewed. Although this is a time-saver, sometimes the renewal continues long after it was needed. I interviewed a patient who, for the past year, had been using a nebulized medicine to thin his excessive mucus. Had he read the package insert, he would have learned that using it for more than several days at a time was only going to increase his bronchial irritation. A couple weeks after he stopped using it, his mucus production returned to normal. The medication was probably needed at one time but it just kept getting automatically renewed long after it was necessary.

Another patient with a long history of emphysema developed a URI. After coughing excessively for a week, he went to a walk-in clinic with the chief complaint of chest pain from coughing. Following an examination, he was prescribed an antibiotic to treat the infections and codeine to suppress his cough. That seemed to work just fine; he didn't have to cough for the next few days. Unfortunately, he *needed* to cough. Too much mucus accumulated and he died of pneumonia a week later.

These are just two examples of why it is important to understand any prescription medicine you take and have a working knowledge of your own current medical conditions. Medical clinics, where multiple doctors participate, are quite common today. If you are seeing a new doctor at each appointment, things could be missed. Prior to going to an appointment, prepare a list of questions or concerns. Don't wait until walking out the door to start. Begin it weeks in advance. Include a complete, up-to-date list of all your current medicines and medical conditions. That way the doctor won't be limited to what may be an incomplete or outdated list in the chart. They will appreciate the fact that you're paying attention and are participating in your care.

While preparing the medication list, make three copies as well. One for your wallet, one to keep in the glove compartment of your car, the other to go in or on your refrigerator. Why the car? Following an automobile accident and a trip to the emergency room, is the doctor on duty going to know you? Probably not. That list in your wallet will help them make more appropriate decisions and could be a lifesaver. If, however, that wallet ends up on the other side of the road, the emergency responders may not find it. Police and ambulance crews are trained to look in the glove compartment for medical information. And the refrigerator? One of the more common reasons for 911 calls to homes is diabetic or insulin complications. Many times, the patient and/or family members are unable to provide needed information. Paramedics are trained to look for insulin in the refrigerator—a cool, dark place. If they find insulin, they'll have a pretty good clue as to why their patient is on the living room floor twitching.

I once cared for a patient in ICU who normally had a low blood pressure around 70/40 mmHg or thereabout. That was her normal pressure and she didn't have any problems because of it. One morning, when she got up, she felt dizzy. A little while later, when it didn't improve, she called the doctor's office. They advised to have someone drive her to the emergency department—not to drive herself. Since she lived alone and had no one to help her, the nurse told her to lie down and called 911 for her. The paramedics arrived in a few minutes and by then the patient was so dizzy and disoriented she couldn't answer questions. The paramedics didn't find insulin in the refrigerator, but when they took her blood pressure, they saw it was low. They assumed she was in shock, probably because of dehydration, a logical assumption. Two IVs were started to increase her blood pressure. Unfortunately, she wasn't dehydrated and the IVs put her in fluid overload, further straining her heart. When they put her in a head-down/feet-up position, to treat her for shock, her breathing became labored. By now, she was really in trouble so they inserted a tube in her lungs and put her on a ventilator. She was in ICU for two days before they discovered that an inner ear infection had caused the dizziness. In all fairness, she was treated appropriately based on the information and clinical signs and symptoms available to the EMTs and doctors. Initially, they didn't know any more about her than what they saw. She now has her list of medicines, medical history, doctor's and insurance information in her purse, on her refrigerator and in her car. On the list she has written in bold letters "My blood pressure is normally low—don't mess with it."

For many, sleep apnea and the use of CPAP or BiPAP equipment are part of one's health care therapies. That information, along with the appropriate pressure settings for your needs, needs to be included with one's list of prescription medicines. As a matter of comfort, when you are admitted to a hospital for any reason, ask for permission to use your home sleep apnea equipment. Although the hospital has similar devices, equipment that one is already acclimated to will be better tolerated. And the flow pattern and pressure settings used on the hospital devices may be just be a guess. Although pressure settings higher than what's needed won't be harmful, they may be uncomfortable. Too little pressure and it won't help. Be sure to list those settings along your list of medicines. The same advice goes for the use of any supplemental oxygen. When one is admitted for non-cardiopulmonary reasons, attention to oxygen needs may be overlooked. This is especially true if supplemental oxygen is only used during sleep. Have it listed because oxygen is a prescribed drug and needs to be included with the medication list.

Following is an example of a form that could be used and of course modified to meet individual needs. Again, in the wallet, in the car and on or in the refrigerator. Most fire stations have a similar form called "The Vial of Life" and should be placed in a typical medication vial which is what the paramedics would be looking for. On your cell phone, under the contacts menu, enter ICE (for "In Case of Emergency") and enter pertinent information. Some of the more advanced cell phones have folders that can store additional medical information. Some folks have placed copies of their medical information, ECGs and x-rays on a portable thumb drive, which would also be useful in an emergency. That is, if the hospital computer is compatible with the program used to store the data. Although technology has its uses, sometimes just a simple piece of paper will do the trick.

Handwritten prescriptions are basically a thing of the past. Most offices are now using computerized scripting sent directly to the pharmacy of choice. Although more convenient, typos and clicking on the wrong box can happen. Some doctors call the pharmacy directly; however, many drugs have similar-sounding names. Zantac can sound like

Name:		
Address:		
Home Phone:	Cell Phone:	
Date of Birth:	Blood Type:	Religion:
Known Allergies:		
Emergency Contact		
Name:	Relationship	Phone
Name:	Relationship	Phone
Name:	Relationship	Phone
Physicians		
Dr.	Specialty	Phone
Dr.	Specialty	Phone
Dr.	Specialty	Phone
Known Medical History		
Medications & Supplements		
Medical Insurance Information		
Name & Group #		
Phone:		

In Case of Emergency worksheet.

Xanax, especially when different accents are thrown into the mix. When given a new prescription, make sure you know the name, what it's for, how it is to be taken and how often. When picking it up from the pharmacy, make sure the information is the same. If there is a discrepancy, find out about it before leaving—*don't just assume, because mistakes can be made.*

Another patient always had trouble swallowing pills. Even small pills got stuck in her throat. Recently, a daily potassium supplement had been started. Unfortunately, the pill was about as big as her thumb, causing her to gag. In frustration, one morning she solved the problem by crushing it into a powder. Fortunately, she had a follow up appointment with her doctor later that morning. When the nurse found her pulse to be in the 30s she called in the doctor right away. The patient reported that following her morning medication she began to feel very weak and lethargic. The potassium tablet had been coated so it would be slowly absorbed over several hours. When she crushed it, all that coating was gone and she got the full daily dose at once. Fortunately, her doctor recognized the symptoms and was able to help her out—saving her life. The prescription was ultimately filled as a liquid, thus solving her problem. Even though a pill or tablet is "scored," doesn't necessarily mean it can be broken. Some extended release tablets may be coated a particular way and designed to release the drug at different intervals. *Don't just assume; always check with the pharmacist first.*

For some, swallowing even a small pill presents a gagging problem. There is a better way than just throwing the head back and trying to swallow. When hyperextending the head, the flexible esophagus is compressed, making it harder to swallow. Doing the reverse—tipping the chin downward while swallowing—keeps the esophagus from being compressed. Try it sometime and see if it's easier. Since the center of the tongue is more sensitive to gagging, placing the pill to the side of the mouth, then swallowing, may also be helpful.

Another patient had a bad lung infection and was prescribed an oral antibiotic, but after the first ten days, she wasn't any better. Her doctor was surprised but ordered another course of antibiotics with instructions to check back the next week. He emphasized that she should take them as directed, which she was doing. Unfortunately, what she forgot to tell her doctor was that shortly after taking the antibiotic she often became nauseated and vomited. Although she was taking the antibiotic, not enough of it was getting into her system. What may seem insignificant might actually be important for the doctor to know. *Don't assume that the doctor knows that everything that's going on is okay. Speak up.*

Any medicine taken at home is usually considered a "maintenance" dose. If hospitalization is required, maintenance is no longer the goal. Medicine will probably need to be adjusted in dosage, frequency or possibly substituted with something else entirely. Although the admitting doctor, pharmacist and nurse will be reviewing all your current medications, always ask and verify any and all changes. *Sometimes things get missed—don't just presume.*

If supplemental oxygen was needed while one was hospitalized, it may have been necessary to use several different types of oxygen cannula, masks or other breathing devices. When it's time for discharge there may be an assortment of disposable oxygen masks in the room. Since they're going to toss them out anyway, why not use them at home? Your oxygen requirements are now not what they were when you were first hospitalized. The masks could actually be harmful if not used for the right circumstance. Ask the respiratory therapist for their advice. *Don't take the various oxygen devices for granted. One size doesn't fit all.*

A few years ago, my father had a hernia operation. I called him the next day to see how he was doing and he said the pain was terrible. I asked him what they were giving him for pain and he told me, "Something called PRN but it doesn't help." I then called the nurse and asked about his level of pain. She said he must be doing well because he hasn't asked for any pain meds. She said the doctor had ordered Demerol every four hours PRN. I asked her if he knew that PRN means that he has to ask for it. Apparently he didn't. When I called back a few hours later he was sleeping and the nurse told me that Dad had already "put in his order" for the rest of the day. *If not sure if your care is going along as planned, speak up and ask.*

Although things are all set at home, what about travel away from home even for an overnight trip? Bad weather, missed flights and a whole host of other unforeseen events could extend the trip. Don't forget to bring along a few extra days' worth of medicine. This includes portable oxygen as well as CPAP or BiPAP devices. Although it's great to take a vacation away from home, those current medical problems are going to come along. As moms always say—*just in case ... you never know.*

A major stress factor are unplanned excursions from the comfort of home. The need to suddenly evacuate because of natural or man-made disasters. A good practice is to have at least a week's worth of prescription medicine ready to go at a moment's notice. If you live in a region where seasonal weather events could occur, such as hurricanes or blizzards, have a small travel bag packed with recommended supplies ready to go. Include in this bag at least one week's supply of prescriptions, separate from those used on a daily basis. When an emergency evacuation is ordered is not the time to start packing. For those medicines that require storage in a cool, dark place, pack a small insulated bag. Now all that's needed is to remove the medicine from the refrigerator to the bag. When seasonal weather events are likely to be ended, move those regular medicines to the daily supply so they won't expire. In 1992 Hurricane Andrew hit Miami, wiping out all pharmacy and medical supplies. As a result, supplies from around the country were diverted to Miami, leaving temporary shortages elsewhere. Remember that even though a major disaster may not be happening in your neighborhood, the effects could still be felt. The Boy Scout motto *always be prepared* applies here.

Although taking prescriptions correctly is one thing, being able to afford them can be another problem altogether. A frequent item of concern today is the increasing cost of pharmaceuticals. Emergency departments frequently see patients who have run out of medicines because they couldn't afford refills. One might assume that this only happens to those without medical insurance or the homeless, but that's not always the case. Pharmaceutical companies have to pass on the cost of research, development, marketing and liability to the consumers. As their costs continue to increase, so will the cost of prescriptions. And remember, those pharmaceutical companies are for-profit entities. They're just like anybody else: if they don't make a profit, the value of their stock goes down and they go out of business. The doctor may be the most caring and compassionate person in the world, but if they don't pay the light bill, the lights go out. Therefore, for the sake of argument let's push past the "greedy" corporate issues and see what can be done to help us little guys along.

First of all, make sure your medications are taken correctly. Re-read the last few chapters if necessary. Any medication used improperly will not be as effective as it could be. Doctors sometimes have free samples. Those samples are not charity; they are an important marketing strategy for pharmaceutical sales. Newer drug samples are provided to the doctor by the sales representative. Now, rather than just writing a prescription for this new drug, a few samples can be provided. If the results are favorable, the doctor will be more likely to prescribe it the next time. Use this advantage and always ask the doctor if samples are available. If so, they'll be glad to provide them. Don't, however, ask the pharmacist for samples because they're not allowed to have or dispense samples; only the doctor can do so.

It's frustrating to take a new prescription for a few days only to find out you're having an adverse reaction to it. Of course, the advice will be to stop taking it. An alternative with a new prescription is to ask the pharmacist for a partial fill and to prorate the cost. If insurance co-pays are used, they typically apply to the total amount that's ordered. However, pharmacies are able to break this down to individual doses and prorate the cost. Yes, it's more work for them, and they would rather not do it, but it can be done. Of course, if the new medicine is well tolerated and seems to be working, a return trip for the remainder of the prescription will be necessary. If, however, that new prescription is unable to be tolerated there won't now be useless medicine, that has been paid for, on the shelf. This strategy can also be useful if finances are such to prohibit having it filled. Especially if it's medication that is needed right away, where waiting even a few more days, could make things much worse. A word of caution is necessary here. Most people have a stockpile of unused medicines on hand. Don't be swayed by a well-intentioned neighbor who says, "I had something like that, and this is what they gave me but I don't need it anymore. Here, try it." The neighbor may want to be helpful, but *it's not safe to take someone else's prescriptions!*

Regarding the price of medicine, people are always amazed at what others are paying. Of course various insurance plans have different coverage, co-pays and deductibles, but that's not always the case. The price of medicine, just like everything else in the free market, revolves around supply and demand. This equation is variable and the price is subject to change from day to day and store to store. Be a good consumer and call around to different pharmacies and ask the price. If quoted a better price, it's not necessary to drive to another pharmacy across town. Get the name of the pharmacist who quoted the price, phone number, the quoted price and then call your pharmacist and ask if they can match the price. They don't have to, but they probably will. *They don't want to lose a customer.*

Of course everyone knows about generic drugs. Essentially they are the brand-name drugs whose patent has expired. The parent company invested billions to research, develop and market it, but now that exclusivity has expired. Other pharmaceutical companies now have the right to that recipe. The price difference is because the generic pharmaceutical company doesn't have any up-front expense to recoup. They can sell at a lower price and still make a profit. That's the only reason generics are less expensive. It's not because the active ingredient has been altered. By law, the generic drug must have the exact same active ingredient that results in the desired effect as the brand-name. Although the active ingredient must remain the same, each pharmaceutical company will add different fillers. These are other ingredients added for various reasons. All medicines, brand-names included, contain fillers. Although the brand-name may have been well tolerated, the fillers in the generic may cause side unwanted side effects. To be fair, many have found the opposite to happen, unable to tolerate the brand-name but the generic works fine. In most states, pharmacies are required to fill any prescription with a generic substitute. The only exceptions are

1. If a generic is not available.
2. If the ordering doctor specifically orders "no substitutions."
3. If you specifically request no substitutions.

There may very well be legitimate medical reasons to request the brand-name over the generic. It won't, however, be because the generic is less potent than the brand-name.

I normally take a blood pressure pill in the amount of 50 mg. The problem was my insurance would not authorize a refill until two days before I ran out. Depending on holidays, etc., I would sometimes be out of medicine for a few days. I asked my doctor about a 100 mg dose which I could cut in half (yes, I checked with the doctor first) so refills wouldn't be a problem. It worked fine, but about three days later I noticed a rash on my chest. When it didn't go away, I asked the pharmacist if the change in medicine could do it. She didn't think so since everything was the "same," but as it turned out, the 50 mg pill was made by one manufacturer and the 100 mg by another. Even though the generic name was the same, the fillers were different. In a few days, my body got used to the difference and the rash went away.

A term often used in many insurance plans is **step therapy** for medicines used for maintenance of chronic conditions. As a method to help reduce costs, the least expensive drug option is tried first. If the results aren't satisfactory, then more expensive ones will be authorized.

It sometimes seems that doctors always order the most expensive medicines. Most likely, though, they don't have any realistic idea what the cost will be. Individual costs vary from pharmacy to pharmacy as well as deductibles and co-pays. The doctor just orders the prescription; they don't have the time to go shopping around for the best price. Whenever prescription drug coverage is included with the insurance plan, it will always include a **drug formulary**. This is a listing of all preferred medicines. All insurance companies negotiate the price of individual drugs and place them in groups called **tiers**. Normally, formularies consist of four tiers which will determine the patient's portion of the cost. In general, descriptions of the individual tiers are

Tier 1: Usually includes preferred generic medicines.
Tier 2: Includes preferred brand-names for which the insurer has negotiated a better price. However generic meds that are more expensive may also be here.

Tier 3: Includes non-preferred brand-name medicines that may
not have a generic alternative.
Tier 4: Includes specialty drugs.

Medications may be in a tier 3 or 4 if there is an alternative medicine in a lower tier that does the same thing. If prescription drug coverage is included with one's medical insurance, obtain a copy of the drug
formulary and have the doctor order from that menu. Remember in
Chapter 3 when the different classifications of medicines were listed?
There were a lot of them in each category and they all have a different
price tag. Doctors are ordering medicines from a particular class, for a
specific result. Ask them to order one in the lowest tier. If they insist on
ordering the most expensive one, it's fair to ask why. There very well may
be a specific reason, but then again it could just be that medication is the
one the doctor always likes to order, but not for any particular reason.
It's your money. Ask.

Another patient told me his insurance co-pay was $15 for all pre-
scriptions no matter how expensive they were. He was taking about a
dozen different medicines, so I had him call the pharmacy and ask what
the "off the shelf" price was—without insurance. He was shocked to
find out that three of his prescriptions were less than $5 each on the
open market. Some of these prescriptions are relatively inexpensive. If
you wish to pay the deductible, they'll take it. *It doesn't cost a thing to
ask.*

Some pharmacies, especially ones in supermarkets or the big-box
stores, even offer a few prescriptions on a no-cost basis. Again, it's not
because they want to be good guys, it's business. While waiting for the
prescription to be filled, you'll probably go shopping there as well. Ever
wonder why they often quote a wait time of 20 minutes? That's short
enough so as not to be discouraging but long enough to allow for some
shopping. Business is business, so take advantage of it. Those larger discount clubs that require membership dues also offer substantial discounts on many prescriptions. Membership is not required to use their
pharmacy. That's because they sell to government-subsidized programs
such as Medicare. They, therefore, by federal law, must make these
same benefits available to everyone. Of course, shopping in the rest of
the store is for members only. *But take advantage of those pharmacy
discounts.*

Pharmaceutical companies know that patients who use one type of
medicine will likely have to use another for related reasons. As a matter of convenience, several medicines may be combined into one, which
could be an advantage if you are paying co-pays. However, be careful; it

could be more expensive than you wish if two inexpensive (generic) prescriptions are now combined into a more expensive brand-name product. *When in doubt, ask the pharmacist for the best price.*

All pharmaceutical companies (the ones who actually make the medication) offer **patient assistant programs**. In some cases, purchases can be made directly from the manufacturer, at a steep discount or sometimes at no cost. Now that's awfully nice of them, but actually it's just business. Again it's back to supply and demand. All medications have expiration dates. If there is a large supply that will soon expire, it's more profitable to reduce the cost or give it away for a full tax credit. Otherwise they'll end up throwing them away. Ask the pharmacist for the name of the manufacturer and the 800 toll-free number. If your medicine is on their list, they'll help with the necessary steps. If your medication is not on the current list, don't be discouraged, what is not available one month may be available at a later date. *It's a toll-free call and the worst they can say is no.*

When shopping for prescription drug coverage, it is well worth the effort to shop around. Some plans advertise free or very low co-pays and deductibles. However, if one isn't using any of those medicines, it won't be very helpful. If you have numerous prescriptions, try to select a plan that covers the most expensive ones. Some discount coupons might be available at the pharmacy, which could save some money; just ask. *Be a good shopper.*

Many prescriptions are now delivered via mail order. Normally a three-month supply will be shipped. The initial cost may be higher but overall costs should be less. Many insurance plans pass the savings along if their designated mail-in pharmacy is used. This should be for maintenance medication, the ones that are expected to be needed for an extended period of time. In the United States, the free market will dictate the price, which will change by whatever the market will bear. In other countries—Canada, for example—the cost of pharmaceuticals is set and controlled by the government. Therefore, any pharmaceutical company wishing to do business there must comply with all price restrictions.

These are just a few suggestions that could be helpful when you are faced with the high cost of prescription medicines. Remember, though, that each community often has additional resources available to help. *Don't be embarrassed or afraid to ask. Be a good shopper.*

The last three chapters have covered different aspects of prescription COPD and asthma medicines. There is still one to be covered, perhaps the most important one of all: oxygen. Not every patient with chronic lung disease will need supplemental oxygen, but if it's needed, nothing else will do. Let's take a deep breath and see what the next chapter has to offer.

Additional Reading

Michael W. Smith, MD, 2 September 2020, "Patient Assistance Programs for Prescriptions," www.webMD.com.
Debra Sullivan, PhD, MSW, 20 March 2019, "How to Swallow a Pill: 8 Methods Worth Trying," www.healthline.com.
"6 Ways to Help with Prescription Costs," www.medicare.gov.

6

What's the Deal
with Oxygen?

Dyspnea is the medical term for shortness of breath and is a **subjective measurement**. Subjective means "how it feels to you." Usually dyspnea means that the amount of oxygen in the blood is lower than it should be. Although routine testing can measure this, it still doesn't define dyspnea. What feels like shortness of breath to one person may not be the same to someone else. Although there are many situations that will cause the sensation of dyspnea, it's the patient who is treated, not just the numbers. When you come into the emergency department complaining of shortness of breath, chest pain or any number of similar ailments, oxygen will likely be one of the first "drugs" administered. An oxygen mask or nasal cannula will be used to quickly increase the percentage of inhaled oxygen. The device used will depend on your immediate needs and will be adjusted depending on the response. Dyspnea can be the result of any number of things and is very often a combination of several. However, identifying the cause may take a while, so first things first; we'll administer oxygen and you "go with the flow," so to speak. Just get your breath back, then we'll talk.

Several different apparatuses may be used to provide supplemental oxygen. The device used and flow rates selected will be based on clinical symptoms. Adjustments will be made as conditions warrant.

Nasal cannula is the most common device used. Two short prongs are placed in the nostrils to administer oxygen. In the hospital setting two types of nasal cannula are commonly used:

1. **Regular nasal cannula**, which is suitable for 100% oxygen flows around 5 liters per minute (LPM) or less. The exact oxygen percentage is variable, since room air is entrained and mixed along with the oxygen. The nasal cannula will be effective even if one is also breathing through the mouth.

2. **High-flow cannula**, which appears similar to a regular cannula, however, is constructed to allow substantially higher flows, up to 60 LPM. Normally this style is attached to an oxygen blender capable of regulating the percentage of oxygen delivered up to 100%. Due to the high flow rates, these cannulas are often heated and humidified.

Oxygen masks may be used depending on clinical conditions.

1. **Simple oxygen mask.** This mask is fitted over the nose and mouth. This configuration is without a reservoir bag or one-way-valves. Flow rates should be at least 5 LPM to adequately wash out expired carbon dioxide. Generally, they provide slightly higher oxygen concentrations, since less room air is able to be entrained during inhalation.
2. A **non-rebreathing mask** (NRM) has a reservoir bag attached that is filled with oxygen. One-way valves on each side prevent room air from being inhaled but allow for venting of exhalation. Another valve between the mask and reservoir bag prevents exhalation back into the bag. Flow rates must be sufficient to keep the reservoir bag full (not collapsed when inhaling), since the flow of oxygen is providing the total inspired gas.
3. **Partial re-breathing mask.** This mask looks similar to the NRM; however, all three valves have been removed. This configuration allows a small amount of exhaled air to enter the reservoir and be re-breathed. Normally carbon dioxide is the stimulus to breathe, and this application may stimulate breathing and reverse dyspnea. However, patients with COPD often already have elevated levels of carbon dioxide and this configuration could be dangerous.

Venti-Mask: This specialized mask mixes the oxygen flow along with entrained room air before it reaches the mask. As a result, a precise concentration of oxygen is attained while a high flow of gas is provided to the patient. Concentrations are determined by various adaptors attached to the large-bore tubing. This style is beneficial for patients with COPD. Oxygen concentrations from 24% up to 50% are possible.

The important thing about these various oxygen devices is that each is used for a specific purpose. What may be necessary in one circumstance may be unsafe in a different situation. As noted, when leaving the hospital, don't take used oxygen equipment home; leave those decisions to the doctor or therapist.

When you are admitted to the emergency department in respiratory distress, the doctor may order an **arterial blood gases (ABG) test** to assess breathing. The ABGs are in the blood coming directly from the heart and lungs before going to the rest of the body. As a result, the ABG test provides a good estimation how well the lungs are working at that particular moment. The customary vital signs of heart rate and blood pressure will also help assess the level of distress. A probe placed on a finger to measure the percentage of oxygen in the blood is called a **pulse oximeter (POX)**. The probe is non-invasive (no blood draw), which makes it ideal for a quick assessment as well as for extended real-time monitoring. What's the difference between the POX and ABG and how are they related? The air we breathe contains an assortment of gases, oxygen being one of them. Although we commonly think of air as "nothing," it does have physical properties such as mass. The weight (mass) of all the gases in the atmosphere is termed **barometric pressure**. At sea level the weight of all that air exerts a pressure of 14.7 lbs. per square inch. Air within the body balances out against this external pressure so it's not really noticed, but it's there. For any one particular gas, that pressure is described as the **partial pressure**, since it represents only a part of the total pressure. The more tightly packed the individual molecules are, the greater the pressure of that particular gas. Inhaled air travels to the alveoli, where it is separated from circulating blood by a thin membrane. The pressure difference between gas in the alveoli and blood creates a **pressure gradient**. In nature, flow goes from higher pressures to lower pressures. The bigger the difference, the better the flow. This difference causes oxygen to move from the alveoli and become **dissolved** in the liquid portion of the blood. The partial pressure of oxygen is described as PO_2 (or in the artery as PaO_2) However, oxygen is not efficiently transported while dissolved in the blood. The importance of the dissolved oxygen is the pressure gradient, which pushes the oxygen molecule onto the hemoglobin of the RBC. This combination of oxygen and hemoglobin is referred to as **oxyhemoglobin**, which efficiently transports the oxygen throughout the body. Although not all variables are represented in the adjacent graph, it illustrates the relationship between dissolved and combined oxygen: The bottom axis (X), represents the partial pressure (PO_2) of **dissolved** oxygen in the blood. The vertical axis (Y) represents the percentage of **combined** oxygen on the hemoglobin. Normally the PO_2 (bottom scale) should be between 80 and 100 mmHg, while the percentage (vertical scale) should be 95–100%. However, when the percentage falls much below 90%, things become a little iffier. Even though the difference in oxygen-carrying capacity between 90 and 100% is minimal, beyond that point, the drop is substantial. That's why an oxygen saturation of around 90% may be reason to begin supplemental oxygen. Because the further down the slope it goes, the more quickly a distressful situation can become serious. The drop down can occur within a few minutes, but the ability to climb back up the hill requires increased work of breathing and takes much longer.

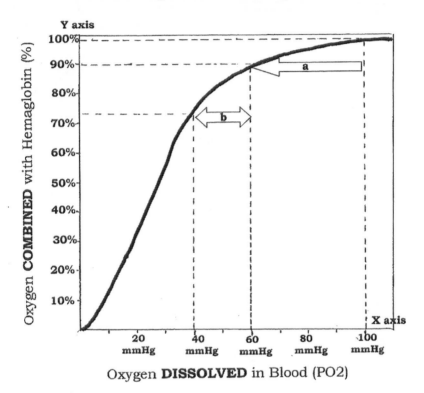

Dissolved vs. combined oxygen.

Basically, there are two situations in which low oxygen levels may cause dyspnea: conditions external to the body and conditions within the body.

Factors External to the Body (i.e., Weather)

Temperature, moisture and circulating air have an impact on the body's ability to breathe. Everyone has preferences as to individual comfort levels. That's why someone is always fiddling with the thermostat. What may be comfortable to one may have the opposite effect for someone else. Usually, it's the extreme or sudden changes in atmospheric conditions that influence breathing. Although we can't change the weather, being aware of its effects can be helpful in planning activities and adapting to the changes. Let's look at a few of these variables.

Barometric pressure: The pressures in the air surrounding Earth are influenced by altitude, moisture and temperature. Since these conditions are not uniform the weather is constantly on the move. Meteorologists predict the weather by monitoring the locations of high- and low-pressure systems. Generally, high pressure brings in fair weather and low pressures are likely to bring the storms. Extreme low pressures are responsible for hurricanes and tornados. During these violent storms, buildings literally explode from within due to the tremendous differences in air pressure gradients indoors and outdoors.

At higher elevations, the canopy of air has less weight, therefore less pressure. The oxygen molecules are still there, but since the pressure is less, they have moved farther apart (become less dense). As a result, each breath will contain fewer molecules of oxygen, requiring an increased rate and/or depth of breathing. Again, it's the reduced pressure gradient causing the problem. That's why for travelers to the mountains above 8,000–10,000 feet or so, shortness of breath is not uncommon.

At a more modest elevation, the effects of a falling barometric pressure will likely be tolerated without problems. One may experience a little more fatigue than normal but otherwise be able to compensate, but the effects will nevertheless be there. Watch the weather forecast and, if possible, avoid planning strenuous projects during periods of falling barometric pressure. Work smarter, not harder.

Circulating air: Some patients prefer a fan blowing on them constantly, while for others, it's more irritating than helpful. Moving air does not provide more oxygen, although for those desperately short of breath, if it helps, use it. It's common knowledge that changes in the seasons are more likely to be windy. In the spring, when pollen is being released, or autumn, when dried leaves are blowing around, bronchial irritations are likely to exacerbate asthmatic symptoms. During seasonal changes, when first activating ducted heating or air-conditioning systems, accumulated dust will be blown into the home. Annual duct cleaning can reduce the irritation. In the spring, before opening windows for the first time, use a garden hose to clean the screens of accumulated debris. Newer homes are more tightly constructed because of energy conservation regulations. As a result, room air exchange is reduced and the potential for irritation from fumes, dust and mold may present more problems.

Heat and cold: Extreme heat or cold always increase stress to the body. The need to maintain a normal body core temperature is absolutely necessary for survival. Breathing is also a factor in temperature regulation. Air is exhaled at body temperature, while inhaled air needs to absorb body heat. As the environmental temperature increases, vasodilatation and perspiration help to radiate excess body heat. However, when the air temperature comes to within about 15 degrees of normal body temperature (98.6), radiating excess heat is less efficient. Therefore, when the air temperature is in the 90s, breathing plays a larger role. Just look at a shaggy dog on a hot summer day, tongue hanging out and panting. It isn't having trouble breathing; it's just trying to keep cool by ventilating excessive body heat. Unfortunately, the increased work of breathing generates more body heat. Although this is not very efficient, it's what the brain is programmed to do. Therefore, in extreme hot weather, shortness of breath is a common complaint. Not necessarily due to lack of oxygen but rather the need for thermal regulation.

Mildly cooler temperatures tend to increase the density of gases, making it easier to breathe. Extreme cold, however, may cause muscles to spasm (shivering) and expend energy to generate body heat. Sudden changes to extreme cold, such as exiting a warm house into frosty winter air, often generate airway spasms. In such cases, using a scarf to cover the nose and mouth to retain warm exhalations may be helpful.

Humidity: Once again, it's the extremes that are problematic: When it's hot, the air is capable of holding more moisture, which displaces the density of oxygen molecules. The net change is minor, since the body naturally adds water vapor to every inhaled breath. The increased moisture, however, slightly increases the resistance of airflow through the airways, increasing the work of breathing. Add in the increased energy expenditure to regulate the core temperature and humidity becomes a factor. Probably more important, though, increased moisture is capable of carrying more particulates such as dust and other airborne allergens. Very dry air is also a factor because excessive dryness will cause irritation to the bronchial mucosal membranes. This can cause excessive coughing, wheezing and shortness of breath. All in all, even though one can't change the weather, it's an important factor in regulating how we're feeling as well as breathing.

Factors Internal to the Body

Restrictions to ventilation: Any condition that limits the ability to inhale fully. This could be the result of a disease-causing stiffness of the lung or even, in the absence of lung disease, broken ribs or extreme obesity. It's like having a heavy weight on the chest and being unable to take a deep breath.

Obstruction to airflow: Any condition that limits the ability to exhale fully. Excessive pulmonary secretions or narrowing of the bronchial tubes will obstruct flow in both directions.

Diffusion interference: Any condition that slows the movement of oxygen and carbon dioxide between the alveoli and blood will affect breathing. Thickening of the alveoli membrane or alveoli filled with fluid or pus will slow down the movement of these gases. For example, if a glass of water is poured into a paper bag; water dribbles out. If, however, a dozen paper bags are combined into one, the water will still dribble out but it will take longer.

Transport of gases: Although the lungs normally get the blame, dyspnea is often one of the early symptoms of cardiovascular disease. The lungs, heart, blood vessels and blood all must work together. If the heart is irregular the ability to adequately pump blood and transport oxygen will be reduced. If there are too few RBCs with sufficient hemoglobin to accept the oxygen molecule, transport will be affected.

Supply and demand discrepancy: This is something all of us have

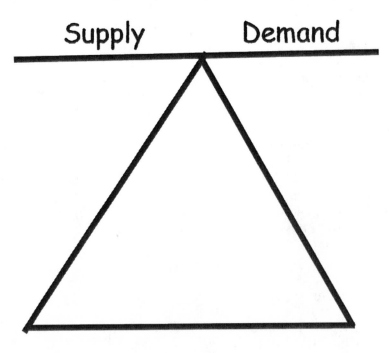

Supply vs. demand scale.

experienced from time to time, lung disease or not. Oxygen is one of the two fuels that the body uses to make muscles and organs work. The other fuel comes from the foods that are consumed and broken down as calories. Even at rest, calories and oxygen are used to release energy. When one begins to walk, energy demands are increased. Heart rate, blood pressure and breathing are all increased to maintain the supply side of the scale. As the walk becomes more brisk, or stairs are climbed, the demand is increased, which must be matched on the supply side. Even though there are a number of things that could enter into this equation, it still comes down to one simple formula: When activity increases to the point where demand exceeds supply, the demand side must be reduced to balance the scale. In other words, one has to stop and catch one's breath. However, when dyspnea persists it's time to find out why and try to correct the cause. When one is coming into the emergency department, the demands (activity) have probably been reduced as much as possible but still not enough. The first order of business then is to increase the supply—we're going to administer some oxygen and see how you do.

Even though the additional oxygen will help, the doctors still need to determine what disrupted the normal equilibrium in the first place. For instance, perhaps a pneumonia has made "marginal" breathing even worse. A few minutes of supplemental oxygen should quickly get things back to normal. And although proper treatment will likely make things better, it won't happen overnight. Supplemental oxygen may be needed for a few days until the infection is brought under control. Without it, the continued respiratory effort will further cause stress to the body and slow the healing process.

When oxygen is needed, one of the first concerns, spoken or unspoken, is "I don't want to get hooked on oxygen." Well, of course not, but it doesn't work that way. The body simply needs a sufficient amount of oxygen, and when supplemental oxygen is needed, it will not increase the need. Many people equate supplemental oxygen use with wearing the pair of reading glasses that initially helped but later were needed all the time. With the glasses, the muscles of the eye didn't need to be flexed as much to focus and gradually became weakened. This isn't the case with the lungs. Once air reaches the alveoli, the gases move across this thin membrane into the blood passively due to the pressure gradient. Using supplemental oxygen won't make the lungs weaker and it will not cause a craving for more oxygen.

If supplemental oxygen is needed, don't remove it in order to walk to the bathroom. Remember the supply/demand scenario: Walking will increase demands as oxygen levels (supply) begin to decrease. A decreased oxygen level is likely to disrupt balance, increasing the likelihood of falls. Don't short the supply side while increasing the demand side. Portable units can be easily carried. If you are hospitalized, have the nurse attach an extension tube to reach the bathroom. Just be careful not to shut the door on the tubing. When you need to be transported to another department for testing or a procedure, make sure portable oxygen is used. Sure, it'll only take a few minutes to get there, but what if there's a delay in transit? That routine trip could easily become an emergency. Better to have it and not need it than the other way around. Insist that they bring it along.

There may come a time when the doctor recommends that oxygen be used at home. Must you be stuck at home, and does the house have to look like an ICU with a bunch of huge ugly tanks sitting around? Is there any common ground here? Of course there is. Technology has helped make it easier to have home oxygen and, better yet, to make it more portable so one need not be homebound. Let's look at the next chapter for a few options.

Additional Reading

Mary Burns, RN, BS, 2 November 2020, "Pulse Oximeters and Oxygen Saturations," www.perf2ndwind.org.
"Oxygen Saturation," 6 October 2020, en.wikipedia.org.
"Oxygen Delivery Systems," 18 February 2020, www.straightanursingstudent.com.

7

Will I Always Have to Haul This O₂ Tank Around with Me?

Just because one has chronic lung disease doesn't mean supplemental oxygen will be required. However, if the doctor deems it necessary, there's no substitute. Fortunately, there are a lot more options available today than in the past, so it's not as cumbersome as it once was. However, one must be aware of those options that are available. The doctor may be aware of your medical needs but is probably unaware of your lifestyle needs. It's important to communicated those needs to the doctor.

First of all, oxygen is a drug and as such needs to be prescribed by a doctor. However, it's not as easy as just taking the prescription to the pharmacy and having it filled. If insurance is involved, they won't pay for it just because a doctor orders it. The insurance company needs proof that it is needed. The requirements may vary depending on individual insurance carriers. The ordering doctor will know the latest requirements and perform the appropriate tests and complete the required documentation. Most likely this will require a supervised six-minute-walk test to monitor your oxygen levels. If you are qualified for supplemental oxygen, a **durable medical equipment (DME)** provider who accepts that insurance plan will then be contacted by the ordering doctor. Once oxygen is delivered to the home, the provider will set it up and explain its operation. Depending on what's ordered, the equipment brought to the home will be one of three types: compressed oxygen in a cylinder, liquid oxygen or an oxygen concentrator, or a combination of these. Let's look at the pros and cons of each.

An *oxygen cylinder* is a cylinder of pure oxygen that has been compressed to around 2000 psi. A **regulator** is applied to the top of the cylinder. It adjusts (regulates) the high pressure down to a usable flow that has been prescribed by the doctor. The size of the cylinder and the flow rate used will determine how long the supply will last. Many cylinders now have a flow regulator as part of the cylinder so it doesn't need to be changed. However, some of the smaller cylinders still have a regulator that will need to be changed when the cylinder is empty. It's not difficult to do, but let's take a quick look at how to do it.

Although there are numerous styles, they all work about the same way. There are two pins in the regulator that fit into two corresponding holes in the cylinder. This configuration ensures that this oxygen regulator can only be placed on an oxygen cylinder. It only fits one way, so if it doesn't fit, turn it around. On the opposite side of the pins will be a screw-type knob used to tighten the regulator to the cylinder. In the area above the two pins will be the port where oxygen flows from the cylinder into the regulator. There will be some type of O-ring (usually rubber or plastic) around this port to help seal it once the regulator is tightened to the cylinder. If it's missing, the cylinder will leak, since metal to metal connections aren't pressure tight. The O-ring doesn't

need to be changed very often, but after a while it will wear thin and the cylinder will slowly leak. When new cylinders are delivered ask to have a few extra O-rings to keep handy. If the regulator is not applied correctly or tightly enough, it will leak, but don't worry, it won't blow up. It's easy to tell when it's tight: it stops hissing. On the regulator will be a gauge that measures the amount of oxygen remaining in the cylinder. The lower range of the scale is usually marked in a red color as an alert that the cylinder will soon need to be replaced. There will also be an adjusting knob with numbers which, when adjusted to the corresponding position, will deliver the desired liter flow.

At the very top of the cylinder itself will be the outlet to

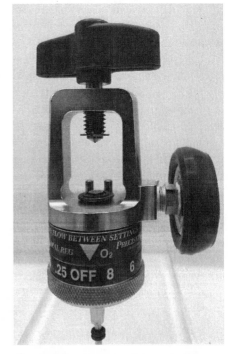

Cylinder, oxygen regulator (courtesy Precision Medical).

allow oxygen from the cylinder to flow into the regulator. Normally it doesn't need to be turned all the way open, but just enough to register on the pressure gauge. Although the oxygen flow can be stopped by turning the regular to off, or zero, it is a good practice to also close the cylinder outlet. Even a very slow leak between the cylinder and regulator could empty the cylinder in a few hours. And last but not least, on the regulator will be an outlet nipple to attach the oxygen equipment. If the regulator has a pulsed-phase system, there will be two outlet nipples for the nasal cannula. A special cannula is necessary with the pulsed-phase system, which won't work without it.

Pros: The cylinders are relatively inexpensive for home medical suppliers to provide and therefore are usually readily available when ordered. Depending on size, the weight of an aluminum cylinder is between 2 and 7 pounds, which can be carried or pulled in a cart. Since they don't require electricity they will still work in the event of electrical interruptions.

Cons: Depending on usage, a number of cylinders will need to be stored at home. Available space could be problematic. Scheduled resupply may require waiting for home delivery, which may disrupt other plans. Cylinders that need to have the regulator removed and reattached when changing cylinders could present problems for those with severely arthritic hands. If using a pulsed-phased system, rather than a continuous flow system, estimating how long the supply will last is a little more variable because as the respiratory rate increases, so will the usage. All cylinders are under high pressure. Normally they are safe to be around, but care must be taken because if the cylinder falls and the stem breaks, the high pressure released would be similar to the release of air from an inflated balloon. Although the heavier cylinder would remain on the floor, the escaping pressure would rapidly spin the cylinder around in an erratic and very dangerous manner.

Oxygen concentrators: Most likely, the DME supplier will provide a concentrator for normal use. It operates as a "molecular sieve" and separates the two primary gases in the atmosphere, nitrogen and oxygen. It concentrates oxygen for delivery while venting the nitrogen back to the atmosphere. It doesn't "manufacture" oxygen and will not "suck all the oxygen out of the air," as is often rumored. Although the operation is somewhat complicated, think of it like this: A compressor pulls air from the room and passes it through a "screen door"; the nitrogen goes through the screen, the oxygen doesn't and is concentrated on the side that flows to the outlet for use. Portable battery-operated units are available, eliminating the need to carry around a cylinder.

Pros: As long as electricity is not interrupted, one is unlikely to have problems. However, several oxygen cylinders will also be provided for emergency purposes. The concentrator is not under any pressure so there is no danger of explosion. All flow-regulating devices are built into the concentrator, so changing regulators is not required. Maintenance is normally minimal and recommended annually by the DME supplier. Battery-powered concentrators are popular and provide a reliable source of portable oxygen. Rechargeable batteries are easily replaced within seconds and are quiet and dependable. Traveling with the battery-powered concentrators is much safer, and they may be used on airlines, which we'll cover later in this chapter.

Cons: Although most newer models are smaller and more energy efficient, older models can be noisy and consume larger amounts of electricity.

Liquid oxygen (LOX): There are three states of matter, solid, liquid or gas, and each will remain in its original state, depending on temperature and pressure. Water, for example, can be ice, liquid or steam, depending on the applied temperature. Oxygen is no different. Normally we think of oxygen as a gas but if cooled enough, it will become a liquid. The critical temperature is around -300 degrees Fahrenheit. When the liquid oxygen is exposed to normal room temperatures, it quickly turns to a gas. What makes liquid oxygen so useful is that when returning to a gas, the expansion ratio is about 1:9. In other words, when that small amount of stored liquid oxygen warms, it expands to a lot of usable gaseous oxygen. The container is essentially a fancy thermos bottle that keeps the liquid cold. When used, a small amount of the liquid oxygen is siphoned into a series of tubes which remain at room temperature. The warmed liquid oxygen quickly returns to a gas and is converted to a room temperature gas long before it reaches the cannula. Due to the extreme temperatures, the liquid oxygen in the portable unit will eventually evaporate and require refilling each day. A larger canister called a **Dewar** will be provided from which to refill the portable device. Depending on usage, the Dewar holds about two weeks of liquid oxygen. Refilling the portable cask is easy, safe and takes about three minutes.

Pros: A full portable system weighs about 5 pounds and is easily carried. The only pressure is the small amount of gas that lies just above the liquid and is about 22 psi. Therefore, there's no danger of explosion. Electricity is not required, so in the event of power failure its use will not be affected.

Cons: Evaporation is the biggest issue, because if it is not used, the stored oxygen will evaporate, which isn't the case with concentrators or cylinders. As a result, most DME suppliers will reserve LOX for patients who require oxygen "most hours" of the day and are active outside the home. Liquid oxygen is a low-pressure device, therefore the only way to measure capacity is by weight. An internal scale is part of the portable unit which estimates its capacity. If the portable unit is tipped on its side, additional LOX may enter the evaporation tubes and freeze, disrupting the flow. Normal room temperature will correct this but it can take a few minutes, during which time it's not usable.

Many of these oxygen devices will be equipped with a **pulsed-phase** or **oxygen conserver** regulator. When in use, this device allows oxygen to flow only during inhalation and stop during exhalation. This conserving mechanism will allow the device to be used for longer periods, which is especially useful if one is out shopping and away from home. To use this feature, a specialized nasal cannula is required. One of the nasal prongs senses negative pressure during inhalation, allowing oxygen to flow out the other nasal prong. At the end of inhalation, the oxygen flow is stopped. As opposed to devices that have a fixed rate of flow, in a pulsed-phase device the amount of usable oxygen remaining is variable depending on the rate and depth of breathing. These oxygen-conserving devices are recommended only during wakeful hours. During sleeping, breathing normally becomes slower and shallower. The inspiratory flow therefore may not be sufficient to trigger the release of oxygen.

Flow rates for oxygen: As with any prescribed drug, the dosage will be prescribed by the doctor. Usually this will be in **liters per minute (LPM)** and is easily adjusted on all devices. Of course, once one has discovered the benefits of just a few liters of oxygen it's tempting to make adjustments. However, cranking that dial up a few notches could be dangerous. Let's review a little physiology. Generally, the stimulus to breathe *normally* is the result of increased carbon dioxide (CO_2), while low oxygen is the backup stimulus. Again, this is normally the case. However, with COPD, the levels of CO_2 are often chronically much higher than normal. As a result, the receptors that monitor CO_2 may not be as dependable anymore as they once were. Many—not all, but many—COPD patients rely on the backup physiology, low blood oxygen, in order to be stimulated to take the next breath. If the flow rate is turned up substantially, the increased oxygen may depress the respiratory drive, reducing the need to keep breathing. Unfortunately, since the CO_2 is already high, it doesn't take too many "missed breaths" before the CO_2 levels become so high that consciousness is lost and breathing stopped. We'll discuss this more in-depth when we talk about exercise physiology, but for now, follow the doctor's orders and don't fiddle with the dials.

Medical oxygen is extremely dry and sometimes causes temporary irritation to the nose and upper airways. It is more likely to happen with

higher flows, but if one's fluids are restricted or one has recently lost fluids due to diarrhea or vomiting, the body's ability to offset this dryness
is lessened. If this is the case, even low flow rates may become uncomfortable. On the other hand, some patients complain of a constant runny
nose when using nasal oxygen. The dryness causing the irritation may be
responsible, and adding a humidifier often remedies this. Ask the therapist if a humidifier is can be added to the device you are using to offset
the dryness. Also, being a "mouth breather" does not require the use of
a mask rather than a nasal cannula. Even when one is breathing through
the nose *and* mouth, the flow of oxygen will be inspired along with the
inhaled room air. An oxygen mask is used for an entirely different reason. If, however, the nasal passages are temporarily totally plugged shut,
the cannula could be placed in the area of the mouth. No matter the
problem, there's always a solution; just ask. Of course, "no smoking" will
be strictly enforced. Although oxygen *is not* flammable, it does support
combustion. Atmospheric oxygen is about 21%, while a cylinder of oxygen contains 100%. That means that in the presence of oxygen, an item
will burst into flames about five times faster and burn five times hotter
than normal. So be careful.

   Traveling with oxygen was once a nightmare, but due to advances
in portable oxygen technology, traveling has become easier and much
safer. Most of us have experienced, at one time or another, the results
of a poorly planned trip. And when medical needs are involved, correct planning is key to success. Let's first of all talk about those short and
longer trips that apply to all forms of travel away from home.

   If supplemental oxygen is needed at home it will be needed when
one is out and about. Better to have it and not need it than the other
way around. Even on a short trip to the grocery store, the unexpected
is encountered: it starts to rain and you hurry and get short of breath.
Forgot the shopping list and it takes longer to find what's needed. Of
course, by now, the checkout line will be horrendously long, as the stress
mounts. And on the way home, traffic is backed up due to an accident.
You're out of breath and the oxygen is at home because, after all, it was
just a short trip. Be prepared. I interviewed a patient who always took
the cylinder with her but always left it in the car while shopping. She
didn't want anyone "looking at her," although, during her excursion into
the store, she always got out of breath, was huffing, puffing and wheezing and had to stop frequently while trying to catch her breath. When
she started to wear her oxygen into the store, she was surprised that
nobody seemed to notice and the store manager no longer had to run up
to her and ask if she needed 911 called. Be prepared.

   When going on an overnight trip, be sure to bring along the medical supplies normally used at home. If oxygen, a CPAP or nebulizer is used, be sure to include them. They need to be considered just as important as any other prescribed medications that would normally be included. Leaving home for an overnight or extended stay is not the same as leaving health problems behind. It's no fun to spend the first few days of a vacation in some strange emergency department. For extended trips, the home care provider should be able to help resupply cylinders or liquid oxygen refills with any affiliated vendors at one's destination or along the way. Just ask. No matter the method of travel, avoid staying seated for more than one hour at a time. Blood flow tends to accumulate in the lower extremities, causing swelling. If you are unable to stand or walk, at least flex your legs and feet frequently to reduce the stagnation of blood flow. Sluggish blood flow does not transport oxygen as well. More seriously, though, when blood is slow moving, blood clots occur more frequently.

Traveling by car: If using cylinder oxygen, make sure it's secured so that a sudden stop won't cause it to go flying or roll under the driver's side and interfere with braking. Avoid storing additional cylinders in direct sunlight and be realistic about the number of cylinders to take along. I once cared for a patient who had been in town for a convention but spent the week in our hospital. He was returning home to Virginia and had 24 oxygen cylinders in his trunk, none of which had been used, which was in part why he ended up in our hospital. If his car had gotten rear-ended, he would have made Wile E. Coyote look like an amateur. Don't over or under pack; be realistic in estimating what's needed.

We've already discussed the effects of weather—temperature, humidity, and pressure—as well as dust, pollen and other pollutants that will affect breathing. While driving on an extended trip, you will most likely be moving into and out of these variables frequently, so be prepared. If traffic is slow or heavy, the exhaust from the car in front can enter if the vents or windows are open. If possible, run the car's ventilation system on recirculation to reduce incoming fumes.

Traveling by bus or train: Someone else is now going to be responsible for your safety as well as the safety of the other passengers, so arrangements *must* be made. Supplemental oxygen *may or may not* be allowed. It's entirely dependent on the individual carrier, so check first. Amtrak does not necessarily guarantee electrical connections for oxygen concentrators. They also require that enough reserve batteries be fully charged to be able to last for 150% of the planned trip. Oxygen cylinders may be allowed, but check first when making reservations. If tickets have already been purchased but their requirements are not met, oxygen won't be allowed onboard. Additionally, the carrier is not required to reimburse the price of the tickets. The need to make previous arrangements cannot be emphasized enough. Another factor to consider: seating is likely to be limited for anyone using supplemental oxygen. It sounds cruel, but in the event of an accident, the oxygen becomes a liability as it may inhibit other passengers from exiting the vehicle.

Taking a cruise: Cruise vacations are much easier now that battery-powered concentrators are available. Most ships will have electrical connections for in-room use or recharging as well as additional electrical outlets in dining and entertainment areas. A medical information form and a note from the doctor is usually required 72 hours in advance of boarding. For obvious reasons, most cruise lines would rather not store a bunch of high-pressure cylinders below the water line. Portable concentrators are the preferred choice but arrangements are still required.

Traveling by air: Portable oxygen concentrator technology has made air travel more convenient now but it still requires a little additional planning. Cabins are pressurized to an equivalent of 6,000–8,000 feet and the change in pressure will affect breathing. In addition to the reduced cabin pressure, a rapid rate of incline can also affect the cardiopulmonary system. These factors may or may not cause symptoms, but if they do, it will be a major problem. The pilot just can't pull over at 30,000 feet. If supplemental oxygen is needed at home, it will more than likely be needed while you are flying. The air inside the cabin is recirculated and very dry, so be sure to drink plenty of fluids. If a rescue inhaler is prescribed, use it when first boarding to optimize breathing before it's needed. Make sure it's kept readily available, and on flights of more than two hours consider using it again even if you are not in distress.

Approved battery-powered oxygen concentrators are generally allowed on all flights beginning or ending in the United States. The key here is "approved" devices, so prior arrangements are necessary, since not all battery-powered concentrators are approved for air travel. If a portable (battery-powered) concentrator is not normally used, a DME provider *may be* able to provide one for your trip, so be sure to ask. Whatever arrangements are made, a letter of medical necessity is usually required and must be signed by a doctor, on letterhead stationery, authorizing the use of oxygen. After all, TSA is not likely to allow a cylinder of oxygen that resembles a bomb through security without proper authorization. Therefore, prior to making reservations for the flight, check with the carrier first to find out their requirements. If they have a particular form that is to be used, have the doctor fill it out *exactly* as requested. Flow rates for on the ground as well as at altitude must also be provided.

Depending on the size of the aircraft, seats designated for supplemental oxygen will be limited so it's highly recommended that arrangements be made at least 72 hours in advance. Some airlines may require the purchase of an additional seat to accommodate the equipment, so be sure to ask. If you are traveling outside the United States and will be making connecting flights, it is important to check with all of the airlines involved. Remember, in outside the United States, electrical outlets may be different, so take along a converter. Sure, it's a little more work now but it will be a lot less stressful in the long run.

We've covered just about everything needed to be considered for a planned trip. However, for those living in areas where seasonal natural disasters such as hurricanes, blizzards or wildfires may occur, additional preparation is necessary. During an approaching event, a plan to "do something" may be too little, too late. The need to evacuate in the face of an immediate threat is stressful enough. The fact that breathing is already an issue only makes it worse. The time to prepare is before it becomes necessary. Although local community services offer suggestions, depending on one's medical needs, additional considerations may be needed. Make a plan and be sure to let friends or family know what you plan to do. During storms, cell phone service may not be available; let somebody know your plan so they have an idea where to start looking for you.

In all situations, it's important to keep up to date with what's going on. Storms, fires and floods may result in havoc for weeks, maybe months. Staying up to date on the events is the first order of business. If you are told to evacuate, do it. Remember, if it's too late to get out, it will be too late for emergency services to get in to help. You'll be on your own.

Most community emergency services are able to offer help. However, in order to anticipate needs and allocate resources, they need to be notified well in advance of who needs what. Each county will have different policies, so be sure to check. Some require a doctor's authorization, other's not. For instance, if they know that a resident depends on a ventilator or oxygen for life support, and the power lines are down, they'll send help to that sector first. It's important to contact the local county administration now and find out their requirements. They usually ask that such requests be updated each year.

1. *Transportation issues*: Although family and friends are normally available to help with transportation, they may be unable to reach you. If a car is available, don't wait until it's time to make a run for

it to get gas. Everyone will have the same idea and the lines will be long. Also, if the power is out, gas can't be pumped.

2. ***Shelters***: Remember that not all evacuation shelters accept pets. If your plans include a furry little loved one, now is the time to find out which shelters accept them. Know where they are and how to get there. Conversely, if you are allergic to pet dander, find a shelter that doesn't allow pets. If using a home ventilator, or an oxygen concentrator that requires electricity, inquire if external generators are available. Again, the time to find these things out is not when it's time to go to a shelter.

3. ***Emergency evacuation bag***: Those small suitcases with a handle and wheels are ideal. Pack several days of appropriate clothing, bottled water and foods that can be eaten as is without the need for cooking. And don't forget a manual can opener, just in case.

4. ***Medication***: Plan to have at least two weeks of medicine available. In major natural disasters, medical suppliers may be unable to resupply their local pharmacies for weeks or longer. Even if the disaster isn't local, regional suppliers may have to divert some of their supplies to the affected area. Order in advance and keep medications with the emergency evacuation bag. If using oxygen, contact the DME to ensure an adequate backup supply.

5. ***Important papers or documents***: Bring all identification cards, insurance information or deeds; any photographs that are irreplaceable should be considered. Many have saved photographs and other documents to computer files or transferred to small portable memory sticks. An emergency evacuation is stressful enough without the additional stress of trying to gather what might be needed. Think these things through in advance and be ready.

Although many medical problems have relatively straightforward solutions, COPD and asthma are different. If a bone is broken, it gets set and a cast is needed for a while. If an ulcer is causing problems, avoiding spicy food will probably help. And although breathing problems can be helped with medications and oxygen, breathing is something only you can do. Let's take a look at the next chapter and learn a few breathing techniques that can be of help through those troubled times.

Additional Reading

Kumar Shital, DO, 26 October 2020, "Oxygen Tanks and How to Choose Them," www.webMd.com.

"Six-Minute Walk Test," 19 February 2020, www.lung.org.

"COPD: Traveling Tips," 14 September 2018, www.my.clevelandclinic.org.

8

Do I Have to Learn
to Breathe All Over Again?

Perhaps breathing didn't start out this way, but over the years, things have changed. Now the dreaded shortness of breath is never far from one's thoughts. Of course, as dyspnea gradually became a more common occurrence, a few adjustments were necessary in order to get by. Ordinary everyday chores that were once spontaneous now need to be evaluated ahead of time. Even leisure activities that were once enjoyable have by necessity been modified or suspended. Lately, invitations to dine out with family and friends have been met with a hesitant response, and your excuses are beginning to wear thin. But what if there's another episode of coughing and gasping for air? What will people think?

It doesn't do any good to place blame on years of bad habits, air pollution or even an unfortunate roll of the hereditary dice. Things are the way they are, and the doctor's prescriptions of inhalers and oxygen are only doing so much. This isn't like the flu, where just taking a few days off and a handful of pills would cure the problem. Sitting around waiting to get better isn't working either. By now, the limitations of modern medicine are becoming apparent.

Fortunately, there is much more that can be done. The act of breathing may now take a little more concentration than it once did, but the alternatives of giving up aren't so good either. To take the sugar coating off it, chronic lung disease is something that one can learn to live with or die from. In the first few chapters of this book the mechanics of normal and abnormal breathing were discussed. Now it's time to apply those principles in order to improve the mechanics of breathing.

The diaphragm is normally used to create air pressure gradients to move air into and out of the lungs. With COPD, and emphysema in particular, the enlarged alveoli tend to flatten the diaphragm, making it less effective. To make up for this, muscles between the ribs, along the neck and shoulders, are used more often. These muscles are referred to as **accessory muscles of ventilation** and are only used to augment breathing when the diaphragm can't quite do enough. Even a professional football player who's just sprinted for a long touchdown will be seen on the sidelines gasping for air and using those accessory muscles. These muscles, however, tire easily and are only designed to help out in times of stress. And what is stress? How about when one can't catch their breath. Now that's stress.

Although a more flattened diaphragm does contribute a little when inhaling, its movement is insufficient to result in an adequate breath. As a result, even minor exertion results in dyspnea. Due to their placement, the accessory muscles are limited in their contribution to ventilation. The muscles between the ribs contract to pull the chest outward against the recoil of the ribs. Muscles in the neck and shoulders lift the chest upward, against the collarbones, to cause the necessary pressure gradient for inhalation. To further complicate matters, this less efficient breathing pattern increases oxygen consumption and carbon dioxide production. When someone is in respiratory distress it's not uncommon to see them trying to catch their breath by sitting at a table with elbows fixed for support, leaning forward slightly while the shoulders are pulled upward with each breath.

During an asthma attack, the airways are narrowed due to bronchial spasms and inflammation, which increase the resistance to breathing. In asthma, the diaphragm will likely be more functional than with emphysema, but the increased airway resistance will necessitate the use of those accessory muscles. In either case, when the demand for ventilation is higher than the supply, the brain calls for increased breathing. In view of the fact that the ability to take a deep breath is limited, breathing stays shallow and rapid, leaving one gulping air—like a fish out of water. Unfortunately, the fast, short inhalations get jumbled up in the upper airways and significantly reduce the flow of air, coming and going. Faster flows result in **turbulence flow**, which impedes the air currents high in the airways, limiting a sufficient depth of breath. A slower flow creates an even air-current pattern termed **laminar flow** that is less obstructive, allowing for a deeper breath. Unfortunately, during those episodes of acute shortness of breath and recovery the natural inclination is to increase ventilation. However, working harder, breathing faster and burning more oxygen drastically slows recovery and adds to already increased panic.

Learning to breathe a little differently is a step that will provide some measure of control and help one recover faster. In fact, with practice some of those acute episodes of dyspnea may be avoided in

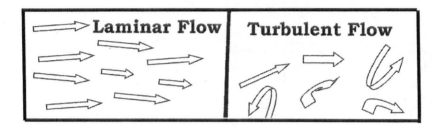

Laminar flow.

the first place. It isn't hard to do and there's nothing to buy. As natural as breathing seems, retraining the brain to respond differently during times of stress does take practice. The good news, though, is that since breathing is something we just have to do, there's plenty of time to practice.

The first step is to slow things down. It sounds backward, to slow down breathing while short of breath. However, air is needed down deeper into the lungs, not just huffing in and out of the open mouth. A technique known as **pursed lip breathing (PLB)** will help to create laminar flow and promote a deeper breath. To do this, begin by breathing in slowly through the nose, filling the lungs slowly and deeply. Once the lungs are full, briefly hold that breath for one or two seconds. Now pucker up the lips, as if trying to whistle, and exhale through those pursed lips, not the nose. The exhalation should be about twice as long as the inhalation. With emphysema, this technique will keep a small amount of back pressure against the hyper-inflated alveoli, allowing for a better exhalation, reducing trapped air. During an asthma attack, hyperventilation tends to dry the airways, which is likely to further irritate the airways and prolong the attack. In comparison to that of the open mouth, the diameter of the nose is smaller, so inhaling through the nose will naturally be slower and steadier, with the reduced airway resistance allowing for a deeper breath.

This technique takes practice, since hyperventilation is the natural inclination when experiencing shortness of breath. Consequently, it takes practice to retrain the brain to resist that which is the natural thing to do. Make a habit of practicing PLB for 15 minutes at least three times a day. Many patients with a long history of chronic lung disease have unknowingly adopted this breathing pattern because it helps, but they never knew why. Now you know. Once this breathing pattern has been learned, you're likely to find you are using it all the time without even having to think about it. Especially before and while performing more strenuous tasks. Over the years, I have observed many COPD patients using PLB even while sleeping.

A second technique for slowing things down is called **diaphragmatic breathing**. With emphysema, hyper-inflated alveoli have caused the diaphragm to become more flattened and therefore less effective. Unfortunately, nothing will bring back its natural shape. The good news, however, is that the diaphragm is a muscle and muscles can be strengthened. And a strengthened muscle always works more efficiently. Patients with chronic bronchitis with excessive mucous and congestion who use diaphragmatic breathing will find their ability to cough improved. Asthmatics will also see improvement as they realize more control over their breathing.

As with PLB, all it takes is practice. Diaphragmatic breathing causes one to concentrate on the diaphragm area and, through biofeedback, practice flexing and relaxing this muscle in order to strengthen it. To begin, first place one hand over the diaphragmatic area, which is located above the belly button and just below the bottom of the breastbone. Place the other hand on the upper chest. During inhalation, as the diaphragm descends and pushes the abdomen outward, the hand over the diaphragm should move out first. The movement of the chest should follow as the lungs fill with air. During exhalation, the muscles over the abdomen should tighten as the exhalation is prolonged because of PLB. Be sure to relax the shoulders and neck muscles while breathing. Remember, it's the diaphragm, not the weaker neck and shoulder muscles, that need to be worked. These two techniques will help move more air with less expenditure of energy. At first it will take a lot of practice to change breathing habits which have evolved in recent years, so don't give up after an attempt or two. With practice, this technique will become natural and will help you regain control during stressful breathing. Although this technique can be practiced in any position, it may be easier to learn while sitting in a chair. It can also be done while lying down, which in fact is an opportunity to practice before going to sleep. While lying on the back, place a book over the diaphragm and watch it rise and fall while breathing. So a quick review of the technique:

1. Relax the shoulders.
2. Place one hand on the chest and the other on the belly.
3. Inhale slowly through the nose for several seconds.
4. While inhaling, the belly should move outward before the upper chest moves.
5. At the end of inhalation, hold the breath for several seconds.

6. Exhale through pursed lips about twice as long as the inhalation and put slight pressure downward on the diaphragm.
7. Repeat.

Diaphragmatic breathing is not a new technique. Vocalists have always used the exercise called "belly breathing" to be able to project their voices to the back of the theater. Pursed lip breathing is also well known to any musician playing any woodwind instrument, since the exhalation is restricted by the instrument. In fact, playing a simple instrument such as a harmonica has helped many COPD patients. It causes the diaphragm to be flexed while one breathes in through the reed valves. Slight back pressure is applied to the overstretched alveoli while exhaling. An added benefit to the harmonica is that the sound can serve as a biofeedback incentive to help when learning these techniques. Additionally, learning to play the harmonica can be fun.

There's one other aspect of breathing mechanics that needs to be discussed and that's coughing. Closely associated with COPD and asthma for a number of reasons, coughing is second only to shortness of breath when it comes to creating distress. However, clearing the airways of excessive secretions is necessary and unfortunately extremely tiring, which often results in dyspnea. Fortunately, there are better ways to go about coughing than just "hacking" away at it. Let's look at the anatomy of a cough, then discover a better way.

When excessive mucus is the problem, there's one fundamental principle that determines success: The amount of air that is able to be compressed below the level of the mucus needing to be expelled. In other words, air must be blasted upward from below the level of the mucus. It can't be gurgled or strained out. In fact, a strong cough will result in a velocity of about 60 mph. But how does one go about it when COPD or asthma has already limited the strength to cough? Here's the anatomy of a cough:

1. Just before a cough, a slightly deeper breath than normal is taken.
2. The epiglottis in the throat is closed to keep air from escaping from the lungs.
3. The muscles of the chest and abdomen are flexed to compress the air in the lungs.
4. The epiglottis is suddenly opened allowing the compressed air to blast out.

Try it and note the steps while doing it. That's a lot of things to coordinate. Unfortunately, coughing usually isn't a one-act play; that one cough gets replayed over and over again until dyspnea or fatigue necessitate stopping. Especially those early morning coughing jags when one first arises. There is a better way to go about it with less effort. Again, it's back to body mechanics.

A good effective cough can be compared to getting ketchup out of the bottle. Good thick ketchup is harder to get out of the bottle than the cheaper thin stuff. Mucus that is drier will be thicker and it will take more energy to expel it. This is one of the factors why the early morning coughing is so difficult. Therefore, proper hydration is essential, not just first thing in the morning, but all day. Now let's look at the ketchup bottle. Those older bottles, with the thin neck, always required more shaking and slapping than the newer styles with the larger diameter neck. If a bronchodilator is prescribed, have it by the bedside and use it when first getting up. Not so much for shortness of breath but rather to increase the diameter of the airways. That way more air will be able to get down past the mucus. That's step 1.

Now let's try to improve the compression (steps 2 and 3). Sitting is probably the best position for coughing. Keep the feet on the floor and the back straight, not reclined. In this position the diaphragm will not be inhibited during inhalation. With the lungs inflated and as the cough is begun, rock forward slightly while coughing. This will improve the chest and abdominal "squeeze" necessary to compress the air in the lungs. The more air compressed, the stronger the cough. It's important to limit the cough attempts to no more than two or three in a row (step 4). After the third cough, the majority of usable air that had been compressed in the lungs has been expelled. Therefore, after that third cough, stop and slowly inhale through the nose. Remember, while coughing out, there was no breathing in going on. And the longer one goes without replenishing the air that was pushed out, the more likely dyspnea will result. The mucus that was moved up with the cough will not be sucked back down the airways. The cilia won't let that happen. Be sure to recover before starting this sequence again. It's not the amount of times one coughs that produces the results, it's the forcefulness of the cough.

With those stubborn coughs there still are a few more tricks that can be helpful; just consider that ketchup bottle. Many of the newer bottles seem to be made upside down. Actually, this makes sense, since gravity is being used to help the ketchup to pour from the bottle. This same principle can be used to help drain the lungs. A technique known as **postural drainage** may be helpful. Mucus is a semi-liquid, and gravity will affect its movement. Liquid flows downhill, but when one is sitting up in a chair, it's an uphill struggle. Try lying down with the area of congestion slightly elevated. It may be helpful to place one pillow under the hip to provide the necessary angle. Don't be uncomfortable.

Give it about 10–15 minutes to help move the mucus higher in the airways before beginning the coughing sequence. Of course, the steeper the angle the more effective the gravity drainage will be. Just remember the steeper the angle, the harder it will be to breathe. Be reasonable and keep it simple. For example, if the right lung seems more congested, lie on the left side for 15–20 minutes so. The elevated right lung will more easily drain down to the larger airways. Once the secretions have been drained from the smaller to the larger central airways the cough will be more effective. It's also a good idea to wait about an hour after eating before using this technique, for obvious reasons.

There's one other thing that can be done to that ketchup bottle, and that's to smack it on the bottom. That's right, whack it a good one to get things moving. In medical jargon, we refer to it as **chest physiotherapy** or **percussion**. The percussion will be more effective if done while one is in a postural drainage position. Have a helper fold their hands in a cupping manner so that a pocket of air will be trapped in the cupped hands while percussions are applied to the chest. Have them keep their thumb closed tightly against the forefinger so air doesn't escape here. If done correctly one should hear a popping rather than a slapping sound. Wear a thin garment such as a T-shirt, since thicker material will absorb much of the vibration. If done properly, the percussion heard can be quite vigorous but yet not uncomfortable.

A device known simply as **the Vest** was originally designed for patients with cystic fibrosis to help mobilize their very thick pulmonary secretions. The rhythmic percussions simulate the action of the cilia and are effective in helping to remove secretions. Unfortunately, the cost of this device is prohibitive for most. Many patients, however, have reported good results with much less expensive muscle vibrators, which are available in many department stores. Although the handheld or full-chair variety will not be as effective as the Vest, they could provide some assistance.

Initiating even a weak cough requires a coordinated effort of briefly blocking the airway while compressing the muscles of the chest and abdomen. But what if the airway is unable to be occluded or muscle strength is insufficient to compress the chest? During the polio epidemic of the early 1950s, a few devices were developed to assist coughing. The paralysis limited their muscular ability to generate a sufficient cough. A simulated cough was generated by quickly shifting between inhaled high and negative pressures. This technique was also helpful for patients who were unable to occlude the airway because of a tracheotomy. Most often these devices were limited to the hospital or extended care facilities due to cost as well as the need for technical assistance.

In the 1970s PEP Therapy (Positive Expiratory Pressure) was found to be beneficial in opening airways that may have been blocked due to excessive secretions. The devices provided increased back pressure during exhalation. Although it didn't necessarily result in a typical cough, opening additional blocked airways and improving ventilation below the level of the secretions was beneficial in mobilizing secretions.

Much more popular today are smaller, handheld devices which are simple to use, relatively inexpensive and require no additional attachments. They are sold under a variety of names, but the term "Flutter Valve" is a generic description. It consists of a mechanism that mechanically briefly blocks the forced exhalation, allowing a small amount of back pressure to be developed. This back pressure is then suddenly released helping to mobilize secretions. This process occurs rapidly as the exhalation continues. The flutter of alternating pressure oscillations is generally well tolerated. Although none of these devices will replace the need to cough, mobilizing the secretions higher up the airways will make expectorating less difficult.

And then there are those coughs that are **non-productive**. A dry repetitive cough that doesn't produce any mucus is equally tiring. They always seem to begin at the most inconvenient times: while at a theater, out shopping or when trying to take a nap. There isn't anything to cough up, but the nagging cough is still a bother. Although sinus drainage gets a lot of the blame, that's not always the case. Have the pharmacist check to see if the cough is a side effect of any medicines you're currently using. If that's a possibility, contact the doctor for alternative substitutes. Remember, though, that a cough is usually the result of an irritation. Very often, it's excessive mucus, but it could be something in the air that irritates the airways; pollen, dust, noxious fumes or even someone's perfume. In this case, the cough is the body's way of "scratching the itch." Unfortunately, the cough is also irritating, which effectively sets up a cycle: **irritation → COUGH → irritation → COUGH → irritation → COUGH, etc.** It doesn't take long before exhaustion and shortness of breath become the bigger problem. Many have told me that when this happens, they just drink a glass of water; others hold their nose and just bear down. Both of these techniques may be helpful, but what's happening is that that the cycle is being broken: Irritation → COUGH = _____ (irritation not caused = end cough). Try that; pull in a deep breath through the nose and hold it, breaking that cycle, and see if that helps slow up that dry hacking cough.

Even when breathing is a problem, there are still activities of daily living that require attention. Applying the knowledge and techniques discussed to this point in the book will help you in completing day-to-day tasks, essentially working smarter, not harder. Now let's turn the page and learn how to put this information to practical use to help get through the day.

Additional Reading

"Pursed Lip Breathing," 14 September 2018, www.my.clevelandclinic.org.
Anna Nicholson, 13 April 2015, "What Are Some Breathing Strategies for COPD?" www.copd.net.
Vijai Sharma, October 2004, "Yoga for Chronic Obstructive Pulmonary Disease," www.yogachicago.com.

9

How Can I Complete My Activities of Daily Living with Less Trouble?

Dyspnea may not be a factor while one is sitting in a chair, but there's more to life than that. Throughout the day, there are those hundred and one things that still need to be done. Simple things like tying a shoelace, dusting or normal housework. It takes a lot longer now, stopping every few minutes while gasping for air. It's frustrating and upsetting. Is there a better way of doing things? Of course there is. Throughout our life we learned a work routine. Sometimes it may not have been the most efficient way, but that's the way we went about it. Things now are different. It's not unusual that as we get older a few adaptions will be necessary. For example, limitations due to arthritis may reduce the spring in one's step or make opening a jar more difficult. Difficulty breathing, however, is a whole other factor. Breathing is something that's required for every task, essential or not. Rather than just giving up, how about looking for ways to accomplish those essential tasks with less effort? Each one of us will have different limitations besides dyspnea, whether in walking, lifting or dressing. Learning to "use what we have" more efficiently will go a long way to help accomplish those necessary tasks that have become burdensome. An occupational therapist specializes in teaching this very topic. It might be helpful to ask the doctor if a consult would be helpful. As discussed earlier, the mechanics of breathing will also play a significant role in either causing or limiting the effects of dyspnea. Let's take a look at some of these normal activities and try to find an easier way to complete them.

Positional dyspnea: By now it's quite apparent that certain positions dramatically affect the ability to breathe. Nevertheless, throughout the day there may be numerous situations where completing a simple task results in shortness of breath. For example, bending over at the waist to tie shoelaces or pick something up from the floor. When doing so, the diaphragm is unable to descend and is actually pushing air from the lungs. If attempting to inhale while in this position, the breath will be limited, with dyspnea the likely result. Think of the chest as an accordion, pulling air in and squeezing air out. The lungs work about the same way. Thus, if bending is necessary, think through the problem: Bending at the waist will restrict inhalation. Before bending, first take a few deeper breaths; prime the pump, so to speak. Next, use pursed lip breathing while slowly bending over to complete the task at hand. Then when straightening back up, begin to inhale. When one is mindful of the mechanics of breathing while performing this simple task, the work of breathing should be minimal. Of course, that will work as long as the task is can be completed in one breath. What about a task that will take longer, for instance wiping up a spill? Try bending down on one knee while keeping the other knee pointed outward, away from the abdomen. Keep the upper body as straight as possible to reduce the restriction on the diaphragm. This way, the diaphragm is still able to assist with inhalation. Although proper body mechanics will make it easier to tie shoelaces, consider wearing shoes that don't require laces. If possible, use one of those "grabbers" (reach extenders) to pick up things that have fallen to the floor. It's all about working smarter, not harder.

Years ago, you never gave an afterthought to bounding up a flight of stairs. Now, however, those daily trips up and down the staircase have become a chore. Once again, being aware of breathing mechanics comes into play. While ascending the stairs, lifting one's body weight against gravity, the expenditure of energy (oxygen) will increase. Be prepared and take it slowly, one step at a time. Don't try to race to the top before getting out of breath; that will only guarantee it. Use pursed lip breathing to help contain the urge to hyperventilate. The body mechanics are similar to when one is bending over. While stepping up, the leading leg will be pushing up on the diaphragm, facilitating exhalation, so plan to exhale while raising the leg up to the next step. Then while actually stepping up, as the body is stretching out, begin the inhalation. Just like the accordion. If one leg is weaker or causing more discomfort than the other, use the stronger leg to do the work of lifting and follow with the weaker leg. Again, it's all about using proper body mechanics to one's advantage.

Reaching and lifting: Reaching up above the level of the chest also interferes with the mechanics of breathing but in the opposite way from positional dyspnea. Remember that not only do we have to inhale;

exhalation is also important. While bending over, it was the restrictions to inhalation that were the problem. However, when reaching up, the chest is being stretched a bit, making it more difficult to adequately exhale. Before lifting an object above shoulder height, first exhale. Then, while lifting and reaching up, inhale. Exhalation should occur as the arms are brought back down. A lateral movement from side to side can also restrict breathing. Reaching across the chest will restrict expansion of the chest. Instead, try reaching with the arm closest to the object, inhaling while stretching the arm out and exhaling while bringing it back to the chest. In this case, it isn't so much about the restrictions on the diaphragm but rather chest expansion.

Bathing: The use of a bathtub can be dangerous while stepping over the rim. When entering or exiting the tub, only one foot will be providing support. Although this position is brief, it's also when most falls occur. Standing close to the tub while stepping will reduce the risk of slipping. Have a non-slip bath mat in the tub and use handrails for support. The use of soap or bath oils in the water will always increase the chance of slippage, even with a bath mat.

When taking a shower, standing requires a lot more effort (and energy consumption) so use a small plastic stool and sit. If possible, use a handheld shower head or a bath brush for difficult-to-reach areas. Avoid the use of strongly scented soaps and shampoos. A shower will always result in more steam in the bathroom, which could affect breathing. Keep the door or window open and use the exhaust fan to reduce steam accumulation. If using oxygen, it can be used while you're in the shower—*but don't use an electric concentrator that's plugged into an outlet.* Use a cylinder, liquid or battery-powered concentrator, and just keep it out of the shower. The oxygen hose can be looped over the shower curtain. Since a positive flow of oxygen will be exiting the cannula, shower water will not interfere with its use.

Drying off with a bath towel can be very tiring. Instead, consider the use of a thick terry cloth bathrobe rather than toweling dry. Just put it on, sit down, pat yourself dry and be patient. The robe can be washed at the same interval as towels would normally be washed.

Dressing: Have the change of clothes laid out before beginning. Stretchy fabrics or loose-fitting garments with fewer fasteners are easier to don. If having a very difficult time breathing, consider delaying dressing until you're breathing easier. It's still important sometime during the day to get out of the nightclothes and get dressed. Take plenty of time while getting dressed. Standing and putting a leg into a pair of trousers requires a precarious balancing act. Sit while dressing to avoid falling. Plan to stop and take a rest after putting on each article of clothing to avoid getting short of breath. This isn't a race. For many, bending over to put on socks is the most difficult part. If so, it might be better to start with the socks first, while one is rested. When putting on socks, loose-fitting fluffy ones may be easier. Avoid bending over at the waist; instead, cross one leg over the other to make reaching the foot easier. A grasping device can also be used to assist with the socks. As suggested, wearing shoes without laces, such as slip-ons, can make dressing easier. Also, a long-handled shoe horn could be useful. Remember to exhale while bending over. Always be mindful of breathing mechanics.

Kitchen activities: Analyze the kitchen supplies and food pantry and reorganize if necessary. Keep cooking utensils in a common location, near where they will be needed. Prolonged standing during food prep and cooking can be tiring. The resultant dyspnea may limit one's stamina to finish the job. Instead of standing, try pulling up a stool and sitting when possible. Bring the items needed to you and work from there. During food prep, might it be possible to prepare a few additional meals that can be frozen for later use? Planning and preparing a few menus a few days in advance can be time- and energy-saving. Consider including menus that can be prepared in one pot or frying pan. No use cleaning several pans when just one could be used. A cooking wok works nicely for this job. Boiling a pot of water can be dangerous, and pots full of water are heavy. Rather than lifting the pot, if possible, try sliding it to where it's needed. If sliding the pot isn't possible, try placing a metal colander in the pot so the ingredients can be lifted out when finished.

An automatic dishwasher is, of course, a time and energy saver. If washing by hand is necessary, first gather the items to be washed, then rest before proceeding. Soak heavily soiled pans prior to scrubbing them. Use a dish rack to let them air dry. Rather than drying, stacking, and putting them away, can they be left out for later use? Work smarter, not harder.

Grocery shopping and eating: Many grocery stores will display a map of their store. Use this to plan the shopping list and avoid forgetting items and having to retrace steps. Many stores now offer on-line shopping and home delivery. See if you qualify for community services such as Meals on Wheels to supplement nutritional needs. Rather than the basic three meals each day, try eating smaller portions five or six times a day. Eat slowly and avoid more than one item per meal that requires a lot of chewing. Drink the majority of liquids toward the end of the meal. More on this in the next chapter.

Carrying items: If possible, obtain a small, lightweight wheeled cart for bringing groceries and other shopping items home, then wheel items to where they are stored. Don't try to lift too much weight. It's much less fatiguing to make several easier trips than one that's too heavy to manage. When carrying items, keep them close to the body. Carrying a load with arms extended away from the body dramatically increases the work. Let the legs do the work of carrying the heavy load. The larger leg muscles will be more efficient, requiring less additional energy.

Laundry: While using a washer and dryer, try doing slightly smaller loads. Larger loads will be heavier and require more (physical) energy. If using a Laundromat, where various washers and dryers are available, avoid excessive bending down or reaching up. Select ones that are front loading and are about chest height. Be very careful when using laundry detergent as the powders can become airborne and some liquid detergent may have bothersome odors. While pouring, hold the detergent close to the proper receptacle and avoid splashes. Bleach can be especially bothersome; when shopping, look for products with less odors.

Ironing can also be fatiguing due to the prolonged standing required. Try lowering the ironing board to a level to facilitate the use of a chair or stool rather than standing. When purchasing new clothes, why not try to select items that require little or no ironing? Work smarter, not harder.

Cleaning: Prioritize cleaning chores; the whole house doesn't need to be done in one day. Anytime dust is likely to be encountered, consider using a cloth face mask. Schedule demanding tasks for those times of the day when you feel rested. Vacuuming can be one of the most tiring of routine household tasks. Pushing the vacuum away and bringing it back multiple times takes a lot of work. If possible, try using it in a continuous forward, walking motion, rather than pushing and pulling back and forth. More walking will be needed but the legs should be better able to do more of the work than the arms. Pace yourself and plan to do only a manageable portion of the vacuuming at a time, then take a rest.

Rather than pushing dust off shelves with a rag, use a microfiber duster that has an electrostatic charge that holds the dust. This will reduce the airborne particles which could activate coughing. Dust higher areas first, then rest for about 20 minutes or so while the dust settles. For non-carpeted floors, a microfiber dust mop will retain dust and is much easier to use. If a broom is needed, use fewer back and forth sweeping motions so as not to compete with the chest expansion of breathing. For larger areas, a large broom such as a garage or push broom might be easier to use.

Cleaning solutions: Glass cleaning solutions often contain irritating chemicals that can cause bronchial and eye irritation. Use with caution and in a well-ventilated area. Spray furniture polish directly on a closely held dusting rag to avoid exposure to excessive aerosolized vapors. Bathroom cleanings with harsh bleach chemicals have resulted in way too many trips to the emergency room. If possible, have someone else scrub the bathroom. If that isn't possible, make sure the room is very well ventilated. Open a window and turn on the exhaust fan. Liquid cleaning solutions that don't produce aerosols seem to cause fewer problems but they still produce irritating vapors. Although a mask may be helpful, vapors will still get through some masks. When using bleach or scrubbing powders, apply the cleaner and immediately leave the area and close the door. Keep the window open and turn on the vent fan to dissipate as much of the vapor as possible. Then reapply the mask and go back to work.

Yard work: What was once a manageable task may now be more than can be easily handled. It may be helpful to use a bronchodilator prior to this activity, since dust and pollen are likely to become airborne. Remember that the weather and barometric pressure will affect the ability to breathe. Watch the weather forecast and plan accordingly as decreasing pressures make breathing somewhat more difficult. High heat and humidity will also take their toll, so be careful; drink plenty of fluids and pace yourself. If working in a flower bed, take your time and avoid prolonged bending or stooping. Always remember the mechanics of breathing and use them to your benefit. Weed killers are much easier to use than is pulling weeds. But what about working smarter; is it time for a lawn service to handle this chore?

Self-assessment: It's not necessary to run to the doctor every day. But looking for any minor changes could provide an early clue when help may be needed. Do this quick assessment about the same time each day, preferably in the morning. That way, if a problem is noted it will be easier to get in touch with the doctor. Be systematic and reasonable in the daily assessment:

1. *Sleep*: Is normal sleep sufficient or are you tired all day? Taking a short nap is not unusual, but if the naps last most of the day, something's not right. If this has been going on for a while, ask the doctor about a sleep assessment. There will always be days when fatigue is more than normal. However, sudden changes in fatigue could be an early sign of infection. Look for additional newer symptoms such as congestion or fever.
2. *Weight*: Day to day, a few pounds up or down isn't much of a worry. A continued pattern in either direction for several days in a row, however, could be a concern. Fluid retention, with swelling especially of the lower extremities, could be an early sign of

insufficient circulation. Always view weight changes relative to recent diet and fluid consumption.

3. *Bowel and bladder*: Have they been normal and consistently appropriate? If one is not adequately hydrated, constipation is likely. Chronic diarrhea should always be discussed with the doctor. Look at the color of the stool. If color has changed from *your normal*, monitor it more closely the next few days. If normal color or consistency doesn't return within a few days, discuss with the doctor.

4. *Medical supplies*: Check the supply of all medicines; is it time to refill? Remember that weekends and holidays the pharmacy may be closed, so allow for that. If you are using oxygen, is the supply on hand sufficient? Are the rescue inhalers in an easy-to-reach place? And is there sufficient amount remaining?

5. *Breathing*: Asthmatics' peak flow measurements must be done daily, otherwise the assessment will be meaningless. Is breathing currently more of a problem than usual?

6. *Coughing*: Any recent changes? Has coughing been excessive or less abundant than normal? The mucus can tell a lot about the what's going on in the lungs, so examine it before properly disposing of it. The purpose of mucus is to help protect the lungs, so any changes could provide important clues to potential problems. Look for a change in color or consistency from what is normally seen. But what should it look like?

    Consistency: Mucus is a gelatinous, slightly sticky to watery substance, the consistency of which is largely dependent on one's level of hydration. If insufficient fluids have been taken in the last 24 hours or so, the mucus will be thicker. Exposure to dryer air will have a similar effect, but that should also stimulate thirst.

    Color: It should normally be clear or white in appearance. Remember that the air breathed normally contains dust and other particles too small to see. Mucus is designed to trap those particles so keep this in mind and use common sense when analyzing it.

    White or clear is normally what is seen, but a change to a *darker white* could be due to increased white blood cells (WBCs) released by the immune system as a result of an early infection. Again a change from *your normal* should alert you to pay closer attention to other early symptoms such as fever.

    Green or yellow: Proteins released from inflammatory cells to kill germs are often responsible for these color changes. This could represent a bacterial or viral infection. A light yellow could represent that the immune system is fighting a recent infection. A darker yellow, a more prolonged problem. Green however may actually indicate that the battle may be about over. Once again monitor additional symptoms and look for changes.

Red or pink: Strong coughing or sneezing very often ruptures small blood capillaries which result in blood-tinged mucus. On a more serious note, bright red could also be an early sign of lung cancer or a blood clot. However, before starting to panic, remember that the mucus that was expectorated also passes through the mouth. Check first to see if there are any bleeding gums, a cold sore or anything else that might have added the blood to the mucus after it left the airways.

Brown or black: A long-standing history of smoking as well as chronic pulmonary infections are often associated with a darkened color. Again, if observing this on a daily basis this shouldn't be a surprise. Also, recent exposures to excessive environmental pollutants such as smoke from a wildfire or windblown dust will deposit particles on the mucus membranes.

Self-monitoring these (suggested) vital signs is critical to the management of any chronic medical condition. The earlier a potential problem is recognized and acted upon, the more likely it is to have an uneventful resolution. Talk with the doctor about what needs to be monitored and when to call for help. Have a plan worked out. Some doctors may wish for you to have an emergency prescription of antibiotics, steroids or diuretics already on hand to avoid delays. For other patients, this may not be practical. This is where a plan with the doctor is extremely important. For some, glucose, serial blood pressure or daily weight (for fluid management) monitoring may be critical. Keeping track of these values and watching trends will reveal a lot more than any single value. On a piece of graph paper, record the results so your doctor can have a better picture of how their therapeutic plan is working. They will appreciate the fact that you are participating in your care.

The ability to inhale oxygen from the air and exhale carbon dioxide back out is fundamental to life. We can only go a few minutes without it, since oxygen is one of the two fuels needed to run our "engines." Food is the other fuel that's needed. We already know what happens when breathing is not adequate. But does the other fuel, food, make any difference? Of course it does, otherwise there wouldn't be all those experts telling us what to eat. No, I'm not going to recommend a diet, but it's important to pay attention to that other fuel. Let's look at the next chapter and see if there is any common ground.

Additional Reading

"Tips for Daily Living (Asthma)," 5 October 2020, www.mylungsmylife.org.
Denise Mann, 20 October 2013, "10 Everyday Activities to Modify for COPD," www.everydayhealth.com.
"Daily Activities and COPD: Tips for Daily Living," www.mylungsmylife.org.

10

How Does What I
Eat and Drink
Affect My Breathing?

Whenever the topic of nutrition comes up, there's always a collective sigh, "Not another diet." However, this chapter isn't going to be about a diet, losing weight, cutting down on sugars or lowering those cholesterol numbers. The emphasis will be on making the most appropriate choices when making dietary selections. Nutrition should be viewed in the same light as the medicine prescribed by the doctor. Food is the fuel the body uses to perform all activities, including breathing. **Digestion** is the process of breaking down the foods that are eaten so they can be metabolized. And **metabolism** is the process that converts food into energy. Foods have different nutritional values, and a measurement of the amount of potential energy value is called a **calorie**. Essentially, the food and drinks that are consumed become the fuel the body uses to "run the engine of life." It's not dissimilar to the fuel used to run a car. And everyone knows that when a poor quality of gas is used to run a car, optimal performance will not be possible. And if poor nutritional sources are used, should one expect anything different? Of course not. It's all about the choices that are made.

Nutrition has always been important to our health, but during different portions of life, those needs change. What was appropriate at one stage may now be inappropriate. A child needs certain nutrients in order to grow up healthy and strong. An adult, with a higher level of activity, requires additional calories and a different set of nutrients. And as the years go by and activity and metabolism are slowed, fewer calories are needed. With aging, the body's ability to absorb some of those needed nutrients decreases and adjustments are again needed. If a chronic medical problem such as diabetes, cardiac or pulmonary disease, is thrown into the mix, appropriate nutritional choices become even more important. Inappropriate choices can result in malnourishment. Those who are severely underweight or very obese are both malnourished. There is a discrepancy between what's needed and what's available for use. Malnourishment may also occur if sufficient nutrients are unable to be properly absorbed. Fortunately, many cereals, bread and milk products are **fortified** with additional nutrients, making more available to the body.

Over 40 different **essential nutrients** are needed each day in order for the body to remain healthy. In other words, without them good health is unlikely. Obviously, some dietary choices are better than others. Fortunately, that's the beauty of it all, since one can learn to make good choices and still enjoy what's being eaten. It's also important to realize that when it comes to nutrition, one size doesn't fit all.

There's no shortage of experts on what should or shouldn't be eaten. And just when we have it all figured out, along comes another study that contradicts everything we thought was right. There're a lot of dietary recommendations for those with diabetes and cardiovascular disease but few on the subject of lung disease. Does that mean that nutrition is not a factor with lung disease? Nothing could be further from the truth. Let's take a closer look at food as a first step in making optimal nutritional choices.

It's not too yummy to think of food as just a collection of molecules hooked together in a specific way. However, that's the way the body sees it. Digestion is the process of breaking apart those molecules and essentially rewriting those chemical formulas. Different combinations are more efficient than others, while some could actually make things worse. To help make better choices, nutritionists have developed a guide called the **food pyramid**, which shows the various food groups and gives a recommendation range of necessary servings. It's important to remember that these are *general recommendations* and each of us has individual needs. So if the doctor has advised you "do this" or "don't do that," it is important to follow their individual advice.

Basically, foods fall into three groups: **fats, carbohydrates** and **proteins**. A mixture of these three groups is needed every day in order to meet nutritional needs. Most of us, however, tend to eat in somewhat of a cyclic fashion. One day, perhaps a lot of fats and proteins, the next day a craving for more carbohydrates. For the most part, those cravings are the body's way of telling us what is needed. Do we always listen? That question doesn't need an answer, does it? Let's examine each of these groups as to their importance and then we'll see how lung disease fits into all of this.

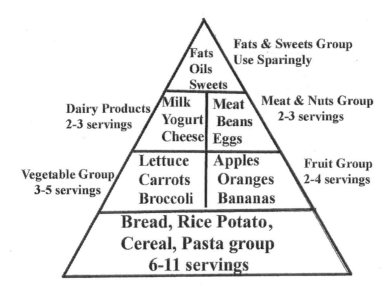

Food categories.

Carbohydrates

At the base of the pyramid are the starches, breads, cereals, rice and pasta. This group consists of carbohydrates and is the principal supplier of caloric needs. Since carbohydrates are easily digested and converted to energy, humans evolved to favor their use. In fact, an average of 60% of daily calories normally come from carbohydrates. It wasn't an accident that humans developed this way. If foods are not properly stored, they tend to spoil. Today, we have numerous resources for storing and replenishing food supplies, but millions of years ago, it was a different story. If an antelope was caught, it only lasted for a few days before it went bad. If fruit was in season, bellies were full for a few more weeks. Unfortunately, between seasons or when game was scarce, starvation was often a reality. Fortunately, our body was preprogrammed to help out during those needy times. Calories consumed but not needed at that time were stored in the body as fat for later use. Attempts to preserve foods were limited to salting, smoking or drying, which was helpful but not all that successful. Grains, however, provided an advantage in that they could be easily stored and therefore more readily available for future use.

On the surface, it would sound like carbohydrates are the way to go. Unfortunately, carbohydrates also produce considerably more carbon dioxide than fats and proteins. The excess CO_2 will ultimately need to be eliminated by the lungs, which is a particular problem with chronic lung disease. While we're on the subject of CO_2, what about soft drinks, or beer? The ingredient that provides the sparkle is carbonation, which is another name for CO_2. Does that rule out dinner at a favorite Italian restaurant, a big bowl of pasta, garlic bread and a beer? No, but remember choices made have consequences, so choose wisely. For instance, if you are just recovering from a bad cold or are otherwise having a bad breathing day, perhaps this wouldn't be a good selection—another day perhaps. It's all about making choices that are appropriate for that set of circumstances. When it comes to carbohydrates, there seems to be a lot of confusion, so let's keep it simple and try to get a better understanding.

During digestion, carbohydrates are broken down to make **glucose**, which is a fuel that gives us energy and keeps things going. It can be used immediately or stored in the liver or muscles for later use. Basically, there are two types of carbohydrates: simple and complex.

Simple carbohydrates are known as **simple sugars**. As one might expect, a cookie can be an excellent source of simple sugars. However, simple sugars are also found in a variety of other foods including fruits and milk. The difference here, though, is that cookies and candies have a lot of added sugars. Simple sugars are easily broken down and changed to glucose. This stimulates the pancreas to release the hormone **insulin**. The insulin then carries the sugars into the individual cells for use. Simple carbohydrates have only two molecular bonds and require less energy to break down and are a good source of "quick energy." The downside, though, is that one is liable to run through this fuel quickly and need to replenish it sooner.

Complex carbohydrates are also known as **starches**. Grain products such as bread, crackers, pasta, potatoes and rice are examples of complex carbohydrates. Unlike the simple sugars, the starches have multiple molecular bonds, making them take longer to digest before they can be used as a glucose source. The good news is that this fuel will last longer. As with simple sugars, some complex carbohydrates are healthier choices than others: **refined complex carbohydrates** have been processed, and during this processing many of the beneficial nutrients and fibers have been removed. However, some of these nutrients may be added back after processing; starches with these added nutrients are called **enriched grains**.

Unrefined complex carbohydrates, on the other hand, remain in their natural form and retain their natural nutrients and fibers. They contain the whole grain and will not be digested as rapidly as the refined products. The result is a more sustained energy release. Unrefined complex carbohydrates are rich sources of vitamins, phytochemicals, minerals and fiber.

Fruits and Vegetables

As children we were constantly reminded to eat fruits and vegetables. That advice remains as important today as it was then. They are the source of most of the **essential vitamins and minerals** that often can't be found in other foods in sufficient amounts to meet one's needs. Essential means we can't remain healthy without them. Far too many people rely on supplemental vitamin tablets rather than eating fruits and vegetables. When looking at the vitamin label one sees the supplement provides some ridiculous multiple like 3,000 times the daily requirement. Shouldn't that be enough? Sorry to say, when taken in vitamin form, only a small fraction of those vitamins are able to be absorbed and utilized by the body. However, when consumed in their natural state, 100% are absorbed. Vitamins are not FDA regulated as a drug or food but rather as a dietary supplement. This means that they do not require rigorous testing and approval by the FDA prior to marketing. Although they are generally safe for use, much can be said about nothing, so buyer beware. Many medical experts agree that vitamin supplements are just fine but they should be just that—supplements taken in addition to eating natural fruits or vegetables—never used as a substitute.

Plant products also produce chemical substances called **phytochemicals**. They help the plant grow and thrive and also protect plants from diseases. Given that plants are living organisms, they are subject to the same assailants as we are: bacteria, viruses, and mold. Basically, all of a plant's immune system is located in the skin. Just notice how quickly an apple turns brown once the skin is cut. When the skin of fruits and vegetables is eaten, we are able to make use of some of those natural defense systems of plants. Much research has been done to show that the chance of getting cancer, heart disease and diabetes can be reduced with a proper intake of various fruits and vegetables. Thus, when eating fruits and vegetables, when possible, leave the skin on.

During normal metabolism, unstable molecules known as **free radicals** are produced. Controlled amounts of free radicals help to fight harmful viruses and to speed the elimination of waste products and toxins. Unfortunately, under certain circumstances, excess amounts have been associated with Alzheimer's, autoimmune disease and cancer. A diet with limited fruits and vegetables as well as exposure to tobacco smoke, pollution and certain chemicals increases risk for these diseases. Fruits and vegetables contain **antioxidants**, which help to neutralize and protect cells from damage from free radicals. Different-colored fruits and vegetables contain different minerals, nutrients and antioxidants. A daily variety of each should be a part of a good nutritional plan.

Proteins

The next two groups will be considered together and consist of the milk, yogurt, cheese group and the meat, poultry, fish, dry beans, eggs, and nuts group. This is the primary group which supplies protein and performs numerous vital functions essential to support life. Although proteins may be used as an energy source, fats and carbohydrates will preferentially be used, since proteins provide so many other vital functions. Fibrous proteins are necessary for maintaining muscles and other connective tissue. Proteins also assist in the storage of minerals such as potassium and iron which are essential in the formation of hemoglobin. They also are used in the development of immunoglobulins, which are a core part of the immune system. Protein receptors located on the outside of cells control which substances are able to enter and leave the cells, including water and nutrients. A diet deficient in protein is often the cause of swelling (edema) in the lower extremities and abdomen. Photographs of starving children show them with distended abdomens, which is fluid accumulation because of the insufficient protein in their diet.

Protein deficiency is one of the more common nutritional deficiencies in the elderly. Consumption of protein-rich food such as meat may be limited due to financial resources. However, protein may be found in various other foods that are much less expensive. Beans, eggs and milk products are all excellent sources. Protein is essential for life, and if it's deficient the body starts to break down, or cannibalize, the muscles to make up the difference. The diaphragm and intercostal muscles—the very muscles that are used to breathe—are some of the initial sources of protein to be broken down. Following surgery or a severe illness, an increase in protein consumption is often recommended to help the body repair and replace tissue that was lost or damaged.

As with the metabolism of any food groups, carbon dioxide is one of the waste products. But the good news is that proteins and fats produce far less carbon dioxide than do carbohydrates. Proteins and fats take more energy to digest than do carbohydrates and they tend to pass through the digestive track much more slowly. Just remember that following a big steak dinner that volume will be sitting in the stomach longer, pushing up on the diaphragm.

Milk and dairy products are important for calcium, which is necessary for building bones and also for nerve conduction. During middle age many adults develop an intolerance to milk products called **lactose intolerance**. Enzymes normally used to digest the sugars in milk are no longer produced in sufficient amounts. Lactose-free products will help to reduce the feeling of bloating that may accompany lactose intolerance. With aging, some of the ability to absorb sufficient amounts of calcium is also lost. Calcium supplements are often recommended to keep bones strong and reduce the occurrence of osteoporosis. And contrary to popular belief, drinking milk *will not* increase the production of mucus in the lungs.

Fats

At the top of the food pyramid are the fats, which should be used sparingly. Unfortunately, fats have a bad reputation in that they are usually high in calories and just a few can add up quickly.

Although fats are an important source of energy, they are also essential to health since they support a number of the body's important functions. They insulate and protect the body from excessive environmental temperature changes. Many vitamins are fat soluble, which means they require the presence of fat to be absorbed more efficiently. However, the problems aren't necessarily with the fats; it's the choice of fats that presents problems. Some fats are unhealthy and should be limited.

Saturated fats are primarily from animal sources such as red meat, poultry and full-fat dairy products. In the body, fat calories that are not used are often stored as saturated fats in the blood vessels, which could reduce blood flow if excessive.

Trans fats occur naturally in some foods in small amounts, but most are made from oils through a processing method called **partial hydrogenation**. This process adds hydrogen to oils, making them more solid at room temperature. They are then easier to cook with and less likely to spoil. Increased amounts of these fats can increase the unhealthy cholesterol (LDL) and reduce the healthy cholesterol (HDL) in the blood, increasing one's risk of developing cardiovascular disease.

Fortunately, there are other healthier choices to be made:

Monounsaturated fats and polyunsaturated fats differ due to the number of double bonds; monounsaturated fats have one double bond while polyunsaturated fats have at least two. The single bonded fats are more likely to be liquid at room temperature. Both of these fats, in moderation, are a healthier choice and tend to raise the healthy blood lipids while lowering the unhealthy ones. Examples of monounsaturated fats include cooking oils such as olive oil, canola oil, sesame oil and fish. Polyunsaturated fats are found in corn oil, cashews, avocados and salmon.

Omega-3 fatty acids are found in fish oils, especially cold-water fish such as salmon. They increase insulin resistance, affect the blood lipids in a positive way and decrease inflammation.

Fiber

One of the few things all nutritional experts agree on is the need for fiber. This is the indigestible portion of plant material, and it's important in assisting with elimination of that which is unable to be digested. Fiber is classified as soluble or insoluble.

Soluble fibers attract water and form a gel which tends to slow digestion. The slowing of digestion helps one feel fuller longer, which is beneficial if one is trying to lose weight. It also has a beneficial effect on insulin and helps to reduce the absorption of dietary cholesterol and lowering the LDL, or bad cholesterol.

Insoluble fibers are considered gut-friendly fibers, since they add bulk to the diet and have a laxative effect. They do not dissolve in water and pass through the digestive tract relatively intact and help to speed up the passage of food. Which fiber is best? Actually, both are important. Recommended levels each day are about 14 grams for every 1,000 calories consumed or an average of about 30 grams each day.

Choices are important but

Nutrition Facts

Serving Size 1 Web Page

Amount Per Serving

Calories 1900	Calories from Fat 12

% Daily Value*

Total Fat 1.5g	**2%**
Saturated Fat 0g	**0%**
Trans Fat 0g	
Cholesterol 0mg	**0%**
Sodium 480mg	**20%**
Potassium 0mg	**0%**
Total Carbohydrate 47g	**16%**
Dietary Fiber 6g	**24%**
Sugars 9g	
Protein 11g	**22%**

Vitamin A 0%	•	Vitamin C 0%
Calcium 10%	•	Iron 15%
Thiamin 20%	•	Riboflavin 8%
Niacin 20%	•	

Nutrition facts (justgrimes).

how do we go about making better choices when selecting foods? While shopping for groceries, we're bombarded with eye-catching advertisements proclaiming "Healthier," "Organic," "Low-Fat," "Free-Range," "Reduced Calories" and so on. However, use caution because the packaging of those cookies may say "40% fewer calories" but that could simply mean there are 40% fewer cookies in the bag. A better place to look is the **nutrition facts label** provided on food products and drinks as well as in many restaurants. This information is available to assist one in making more reasonable selections. Let's take a look at a typical label.

Serving size. Typically, the serving size is based on an average daily diet of 2,000 calories. Important note here: if the serving size is one cup and there are two servings per container and the whole thing is consumed, double all the data.

Calories and calories from fat. Those with weight issues (+/-) should pay particular attention to the number of calories per serving and adjust the serving size accordingly.

Total fat, cholesterol and sodium. Cardiovascular disease is major a concern for much of the population, so these three items are often listed together.

Potassium, fiber, vitamins and minerals. These items are more highly recommended in a healthy diet and are often listed together.

Total carbohydrates, sugars and protein. These are often listed together.

Depending on the product, the sequence of labeling may vary. Remember that these are general recommendations and are designed to help one make better choices in balancing food selections. For example, perhaps a favorite food is higher in sodium than one would like but other foods that would be paired with that meal may be lower in sodium. Using this information could be helpful in preparing a more balanced meal. Regrettably, there's no quick fix with a standard "COPD-Asthma" diet. Other medical conditions such as cardiovascular disease and diabetes may also be part of the problem and require their own dietary recommendations. Always follow the recommendations of your doctor or dietitian.

When one's breathing is already limited, not only what is eaten but when and how are also important. Since the increased work of breathing requires as much as 10–20% more energy, additional calories may be needed. Unfortunately, eating a larger volume limits the movement of the diaphragm, reducing the ability to fully inhale. Shortness of breath results in increased mouth breathing, which dries the tongue and affects the sense of taste; and long-term oxygen flow may dampen the sense of smell. Both of these may reduce one's appetite. Eating may trigger excessive coughing, and during swallowing, there's no breathing, which may increase dyspnea. For some, the energy needed for shopping and preparing meals may also be a limiting factor. As a result, nutrition may take a backseat to breathing because it doesn't seem worth the effort. Let's take a look at a few recommendations that may be helpful.

When you eat: Don't skip breakfast; it sets the nutritional clock for the day, and no, a cup of coffee and a cigarette is not breakfast. Rather than eating two or three traditional meals each day, try five or six smaller portions. This will reduce the volume in the stomach and allow the diaphragm to move more freely. If using a bronchodilator, consider using it about an hour before you plan to eat. Doing so will optimize breathing and help clear the airways of excessive mucus. If possible, plan to rest before scheduled meals. Try to schedule your main meals earlier in the day when energy levels are likely to be higher. This will also provide a little more energy throughout the day. If using oxygen continuously or "as needed," use it while eating.

How you eat: Take smaller bites and chew thoroughly to lessen shortness of breath. Avoid eating while reclining to lessen the restrictions on the diaphragm. Eat slowly to avoid swallowing too much air, which causes bloating. Try to drink the majority of fluids toward the end of the meal to avoid becoming too full to finish the meal. Try eating the higher calorie portions early in the meal before becoming full. When possible, try not to eat alone; make meals more enjoyable.

What you eat: Read the food labels when selecting foods, and not just the calories listings. Select a nutrient plan specific to your individual needs as recommended by the doctor or dietitian. Plan meals that contain some favorite foods, but try to eat a variety each day. Choose a diet composed of the various food groups. Limit simple sugars. Since digestion of carbohydrates results in more carbon dioxide in the blood, reduce slightly the calories from carbohydrates and replace them with protein calories. Don't skip fruits and vegetables; eat a sufficient amount each day to ensure sufficient fiber. Avoid foods that cause gas or bloating. Fried or greasy foods slow the movement through the digestive track and may cause one to feel bloated. When possible, choose foods that are easy to chew and swallow. If fluid retention is a problem, reduce the use of salt, since it causes the body to retain fluids. Avoid carbonated beverages during meals. Alcohol can interfere with medications, especially oral steroids, so use it with caution. Calcium and vitamin D are important to maintain bone health; choose foods that include it, and don't exclude milk. Choose foods that are easy to prepare, saving energy for eating. If you need help cooking ask family or friends to help prepare a number of simple meals that can be frozen for later use. For food assistance, contact Meals on Wheels or other local programs.

Water and Other Fluids

A look at most recommendations offers an easy formula: eight 8-ounce glasses of water per day. Sounds like a lot, but let's look at that a little closer: 8 × 8 = 64 ounces per day, and at 16 ounces per pound, that's four pounds of water each day. For a 100 pound person that's 4% of their body weight, but for a 200 pound person it's only 2%. Yes, size matters. And if other medical complications such as congestive heart failure or kidney disease are part of the problem, that formula will most likely present problems. If the doctor has recommended fluid limitations— stay with those recommendations. For the rest of us, though, ***water should be about half of our fluid intake each day***. It's an easy calculation: Your body weight divided by two. Now, use that number as ounces (don't convert it, just use that number). Now divide that by two again.

Example: ***100 lbs***/2 = 50 Now 50/2 = 25 ounces of water per day
For that body size, 25 ounces of water, or 25/8 ounces per glass = a little more than 3 glasses of water per day.

Example: ***250 lbs***/2 = 125 Now 125/2= about 63 ounces of water per day
For that body size: 63 ounces if water or 63/8 oz. per glass = almost 8 glasses of water per day.

Now that's just water, because other beverages as well as most of the food we eat also contain fluids which comprise the other half of the daily fluid needs. Just remember that caffeinated beverages, such as coffee, soft drinks and alcohol act as diuretics. Therefore, if these choices are more often than occasional, fluid loss could be an issue. Consequently, choices do make a difference. And why is fluid management such an issue? If there is insufficient fluid to keep the mucus thinned, it's going to thicken and be more difficult for the cilia or coughing to remove it from the airways. However, if too much fluid is consumed, fluid retention and swelling of the feet and legs will occur. If not treated, the fluid retention will ultimately back up to the lungs, causing shortness of breath. When body tissue is unable to hold additional fluid, some excess fluid will remain circulating in the blood. This increases the back pressure against the heart, increasing resistance. In the presence of any chronic medical disease as well as in the elderly, attention to nutrition and fluid management is of the utmost importance.

As emphasized earlier, dietary and beverage choices should be considered just as important as the medicines that the doctor is prescribing. A few years ago, I was waiting to pay for my prescriptions. The man ahead of me, who was in one of those electric scooters, was having problems with his Medicaid coverage for one of his prescriptions. It was taking a while, as these things often do, and with nothing else to do I did what many of my collogues do and used simple observation to "guess that diagnosis." The man weighed at least 350 pounds if he weighed an ounce. He wore loose slippers because his feet and ankles were darkened and badly swollen. His neck veins were distended and in spite of the air-conditioning he was sweating profusely. He began wheezing as his conversation with the pharmacist escalated, and when he stood up, a pack of cigarettes fell out of his pocket (which I retrieved for him without comment). My guess was congestive heart failure, diabetes, hypertension, elevated cholesterol and COPD. When his insurance was confirmed and his totals rung up, the name of the medication and price was displayed on the cash register display, which confirmed my unsolicited observations: Lasix (congestive heart failure); Lipitor (cholesterol); Metformin (diabetes); Lisinoprel (hypertension) and an Albuterol inhaler (breathing). He then pulled three items out of his buggy basket, which included a bag of grapefruit, a large ham and a case of soft-drinks. I just couldn't resist a comment and in a nonjudgmental tone spoke up: "Are those items for you or someone else?" I asked. "They're for me; what's it to you?" he snarled. "Well," I began, "I noticed that one of your medicines was Lipitor and didn't your doctor caution you about grapefruit and Lipitor?" The pharmacist was nodding in agreement with me but was sensible enough to stay out of the conversation. "I like grapefruit and it's none of your business." In for the penny, in for the pound, so I added: "I also noticed you're on water pills, and since ham is very salty it will cause you to retain more fluid." "Butt out," he wheezed. "It's none of your business." By now, both of us were close to a hypertensive crisis so I added: "I also noticed that you paid for your prescriptions with a taxpayer-supported federal program and I'm a taxpayer...." Fortunately, cooler heads prevailed and we both backed off before either of us had a stroke.

Too many people throw all the responsibility for their health on their doctor's desk and go on about their merry way and wonder why they aren't getting any better. I once worked with a cardiologist who had a large sign in his office: "Before age 40, God takes pretty good care of us. After age 40, God needs a little help." And that help is a two-way-street with the doctor. If one is not willing to participate in their care plan, don't expect to make any improvements at all. And while talking with the doctor, did the subject of exercise ever come up? I'll bet it has. Unfortunately, that's something that can't be delegated out. You and only you have to take care of that. However, how does one go about it if breathing is already a problem? Not by running laps or doing push-ups like like one did in high school. Your body has changed since then and things are different now. Let's take a deep breath, turn the page and look at exercise a little differently and see how to go about it.

Additional Reading

"Water: How Much Should You Drink Every Day?" 24 October 2020, www.mayoclinic.org.

"Nutrition and COPD," 23 October 2020, www.lung.org.

Clair Janchote, February 2019, "COPD Nutrition Guide: 5 Diet Tips for People with COPD," www.healthline.com.

11

How Can I Start
an Exercise Program
If I'm Having
Trouble Breathing?

When it comes to exercise, it's a phrase often heard: "Use it or lose it." And that about sums up this next chapter. Our body has always been the great accommodator. Under most circumstances, it tries to adapt to almost anything that is asked of it. When sick or injured it is appropriate for the body to rest in order to heal and recover. During this time, the body will quickly adapt to the new level of activity, and muscle tone and the ability to get around decrease. This is true no matter the age or state of one's health; muscle mass and tone decrease when muscles are not used. Remember back a few years to high school and the first few weeks of football practice. Those young jocks walking around all stiff and sore and the smell of liniment was everywhere. In just a few weeks, though, those same athletes became conditioned to their increased level of activity. They now moved with fluidic grace. Those first few weeks of discomfort were necessary to get where they wanted to be. Unfortunately, if an injury sidelined them for a week or so, they had to start their conditioning all over again. It wasn't easy, and it isn't fair that it takes so much effort to get in shape when it can be lost so quickly.

Getting in better shape was easier when you were younger and healthier, but now, with lung disease, is it practical or even safe to begin an exercise program? The answer is a resounding *yes*. Research conducted on thousands of individuals confirmed that exercise is a necessary part in the management of any chronic medical condition, especially for those with heart disease, hypertension, diabetes, arthritis, osteoporosis, depression and, yes, in particular COPD and asthma. The principles are very similar to the maintenance of a car; following a tune-up, it won't run any faster but it will get better mileage. And an exercise program to get one "tuned up" will help make better use of that one fuel that is now limited, oxygen. More efficient use of all energy reserves allows for more work with less fatigue. And work may be as simple as meaning not having to gasp for air when shopping or visiting friends. Exercise improves the ability to get a good night's sleep. Proper rest helps to reduce anxiety and allows one to cope with day-to-day stresses. Exercise helps the immune system function better and reduces the chance of getting sick. Additionally, a structured exercise program helps one to regain a sense of control over circumstances that previously may have been viewed as uncontrolled.

A word of caution, however. Always check with your doctor before beginning an exercise routine. There may be something that needs to be watched closely, and the time to know that is *before*, not later. Although routine exercise will improve one's immune system's ability to fight disease, it will not prevent sickness. Always use reasonable caution and if illness or injuries occur, rest and recover. As soon as a reasonably good recovery is made is the time to get back to a routine again. Go slowly at first, but continue to progress and don't give up.

Most doctors will agree that exercise is always appropriate, only to advise, "Be careful." Where does one start? There's a wise saying: "Before you can run, you have to learn to walk. And before you can walk, you have to learn to stand." So, let's start from there. In the previous chapters the emphasis was about breathing control, use of prescribed medicines and oxygen, food and nutrition. That's the starting point. All those things are important. It isn't wise to just jump into an exercise program without the right tools, and that includes all the things that have been covered so far. Those tools need to be used with any exercise routine. Basically, there are four aspects that need to be considered: improving flexibility, improving aerobic capacity, strength training and recovery.

I. Flexibility: Before beginning to exercise, it's important—in fact, it's vital—to first warm up. Just like a professional athlete or a concert musician; they all warm up before a performance. It's that important. Many people tend to skip this part, and unfortunately put themselves at a greater risk for injury. If joint pain, such as arthritis, is a concern, plan to take any appropriate medicines about 30 minutes before a planned exercise session. Increased activity will most certainly result in the need for increased ventilation. As the airways become drier, bronchial spasms are more likely. If you are asthmatic, consider using a prescribed rescue inhaler prior to starting. Make sure adequate hydration is continued during each session.

There are numerous movements that can be used, but in general, warm up from head to toe. This should take 5 to 10 minutes to complete but don't rush it. The stretching movements should be done slowly with progressive lengthening of the extremity. Don't use fast, jerky movements just to get it out of the way, and don't stretch to the point of pain; it's not necessary. Don't hold your breath. Instead, breathe in when stretching, and slowly exhale while holding the stretch for 5 to 10 seconds. Loosen the neck muscles by slowly turning and rotating your head; shrug and rotate the shoulders and arms. Gradually stretch the muscles of the upper and lower back and of course the legs. Especially, loosen the calf muscles, and rotate the ankles to warm up the joints. These warm-up exercises will not provide the necessary conditioning that is desired, but they are necessary, so don't skip or rush through them.

II. Aerobics: Once the body is warmed up and stretched out, it's time to begin. For those with breathing limitations, endurance-building exercises need to come first before you even considering strength training. Endurance-building exercises are often called ***aerobic exercises***. But what exactly does the term "aerobic" mean? Most would answer that it involves getting the heart rate to a certain level and breaking a sweat. Those indeed are indications of a more vigorous workout, but aerobics has a more specific description. Aerobics quite literally means "in the presence of oxygen." Having sufficient amounts of oxygen in the blood to assist with the extraction of energy from the foods that have been eaten. The bonds that hold the various food molecules together need to be broken to release the stored energy. This process requires an expenditure of energy. Whenever a bond is broken, 3 units of energy are released. If, however, a free oxygen molecule is available to help break the bonds, 18 units of energy are released from that same bond.

It's easy to see that having enough blood oxygen available while performing any physical activity is vital to one's success.

The next aspect of aerobic conditioning to consider is how much is enough and how much is too much? Both are very important benchmarks on the path to improving aerobic conditioning. Too little exercise will limit progress and too much will be problematic. Even the best-conditioned marathon runners will describe the point where they

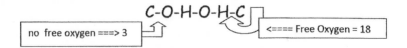

Aerobics defined.

are no longer able to continue as "hitting the wall." With COPD, just walking across the room may be enough to bring one to that point or trigger an asthma attack. Why is it that breathing isn't a problem while one is at rest or even during the first minute or so of walking, but all of a sudden, one's wheezing and gasping for air—what's going on? It's easier to view this in terms of a scale that tries to stay balanced. On one side is supply, which is the amount of oxygen available in the blood at any given time. The other side, demand, determines how much is needed for that activity. The supply side is controlled by the lung's ability to increase the frequency and depth of breathing, increasing the intake of oxygen and expelling carbon dioxide. The heart must also increase its pump work-load and the blood must be available to transport the gas. All of these factors affect the supply side.

The other side of the scale is demand, or simply the amount of work being performed at any particular moment. Factors here may include the speed and amount of incline being walked; also the amount of weight being carried, which includes not only that armload of laun-dry but one's body weight as well. As noted, other factors such as the weather, barometric pressure, temperature and humidity also influence (+/-) either side of the scale. As long as the scale is able to stay balanced,

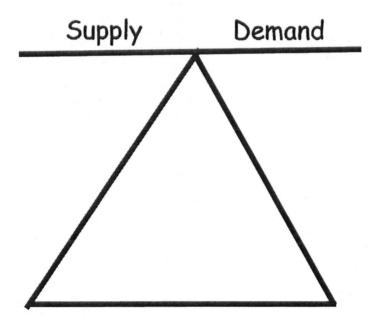

Supply vs. demand scale.

everything is okay. If increasing the demand side, the supply side also needs to be increased in order to keep the scale balanced. As the amount of work continues to increase, one will eventually reach a point where the demand is more than is able to be handled. The scale is out of balance and the only choice now is to reduce the demand until the supply side can catch up. In other words—stop and catch your breath.

The graph above represents the **aerobic threshold** and demonstrates what happens as the level of activity is increased: The bottom of the scale, from left to right, represents time, which could be a brief walk across the room or a much longer event like a marathon. The amount of time it takes is irrelevant here because the processes is always the same:

(A) When one is first starting an activity, the oxygen and carbon dioxide levels are at their resting point of normal stability.

(B) Shortly after the activity begins the oxygen level begins to decrease, since more is being used, and the carbon dioxide begins to increase, since more is being produced. Both of these responses are normal due to the extra work that is now being done.

(C) It doesn't take long for the body to adjust. Recovery begins as the supply side is increased to compensate for the new demands. Increased breathing and heart rate are the body's response to the increased demand and need to replenish the supply side. This is often referred to as getting a second wind.

(D) As the activity continues, things stabilize for a while.

(E) Eventually the scales begin to shift. It becomes more difficult to provide the needed supply, and the ability to compensate is reduced. Oxygen demand increases faster than it can be

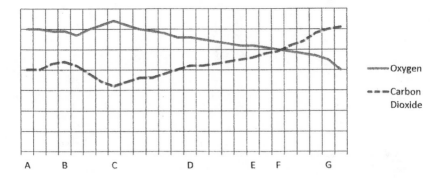

Aerobic threshold.

resupplied, and carbon dioxide is produced in excess of one's ability to adequately expel it.
(F) The point at which the scales eventually cross is called the **aerobic threshold**.
(G) Beyond this point exercise is able to continue but at a higher cost. In other words, only 3 units of energy for every bond broken, rather than 18 will be produced. Although the short-term needs are met, a higher cost has yet to to be accounted for. The apt term now used is aptly named the **oxygen debt**. Repaying the oxygen debt is when one finally has to stop and catch their breath. Until this debt is repaid, breathlessness will continue.

With an exercise program, as muscles improve tone and breathing is better controlled, the aerobic threshold point will be moved a little farther to the right. Remember, this doesn't happen overnight so don't get discouraged. Also, as everyone is well aware of by now, some days will be better than others. Unfortunately, it seems like there are more things on the demand side of the scale to hold one back than the other way around; however, one has to work with what one has.

Our new patient in Pulmonary Rehab was extremely short of breath. The best she could do was walk slowly for only two minutes. After learning proper breathing control and more appropriate use of her supplemental oxygen, with determination, she began to improve. After two months she was able walk on the treadmill for 20 minutes without stopping and she was deservedly proud of her accomplishment. Several months later, a routine physical discovered a cancerous tumor in her abdomen. Her surgeon was reluctant to remove it because of her severe COPD. But without surgery her prospects were also bleak. She had the surgery and, because of her improved conditioning, surprised her doctors and was able to be weaned from the ventilator the very next day. It was several months before she could resume her exercise sessions again but she was anxious to conquer her old nemesis, the treadmill. However, two minutes was all she could do now. Discouraging, sure, but it didn't stop her because she had confidence that she could do it again and this time she knew how. Nobody was surprised that after another month she was back at her 20-minute mark again. There are always going to be those ups and downs. Don't get discouraged—that's life. Deal with it.

The starting point for any training program, at any level, is identifying and setting realistic and achievable goals. First, list the activities that are now limited because of breathing. Then look over that list and determine which activities need to be completed vs. ones that would be nice to do. Next, develop a method for keeping track of progress, a scorecard of sorts. It doesn't have to be fancy or complicated; keep it simple. Motivation is essential when beginning, and any sort of measurement will help determine if progress is being made. Write it down so you will have something to refer back to. We'll expand on this in the final chapter, so stay tuned.

It's important to start out exercise slowly to lessen the chance of injury or shortness of breath. When recovering from a prolonged illness, one's legs will be weak and balance and stability a likely concern. So, let's start from there. While seated awake in a chair, stand for several minutes every 15 minutes or so. If watching television, every time a commercial comes on, stand until it's finished. That way if balance problems or extreme fatigue occur, the chair is right there for recovery. Just using the leg and abdominal muscles to rise from the chair will help to strengthen these muscles. Even in a severely weakened condition, improvement will be noticed in a few days. Of course this is not the final answer. Remember, before one can walk, one has to first stand. Once ambulation is better, progress to a stationary bike—not a regular bike—not yet. Watch yourself progress.

However, always plodding along at the same slow pace or pushing too hard isn't the answer either. Plan to start off with a three-week schedule of at least two but not more than three exercise sessions per week. Take a day off between sessions to recover. Remember, getting out of shape didn't occur in just one or two days and getting back in shape won't happen that fast either. Be patient but persistent. If using a fitness center, make use of the various devices, such as treadmills, bikes and arm ergometers. Depending on the severity of your cardiopulmonary limitations, try various devices for about five minutes with twice that long between devices to recover. Each session, try to add several minutes to exercise times, as tolerated. The goal for the first two weeks should be about 20 minutes of total aerobic exercise each session. Don't limit the exercises to just one type of device such as the treadmill or bike. Remember, the goal is for overall fitness, so use various pieces of equipment. Save weight training for a few weeks later; aerobic conditioning needs to improve first.

If starting an unsupervised exercise program at home, walking will most likely be the primary exercise. Pick out a spot that you are able to walk to without stopping. That's the initial short-term goal. After a week or so, that distance should become easier. If not, reassess the distance and breathing techniques being used. Once progress is realized, select additional "assessment points" to continue improvement. At each point, stop and assess breathing to determine when to walk to the next planned resting point. Be careful not to set goals too far away from the starting point, since it's important to be able to get back home. This is a useful tool when walking in an unfamiliar area, such as when shopping. Before walking, pick out realistic stopping points. Don't just keep going until you are out of breath. Plan it out. If living near an indoor shopping mall, ask about a **mall-walkers** program. Most malls encourage participation and open the mall (not the stores) about an hour earlier for walkers. This will provide a safe place to walk without the cold of winter or the heat of summer to be used as an excuse to stay in bed.

If a pool is available, use that as well (weather permitting, of course). Swimming laps isn't necessary; just walking against the resistance of the water is excellent exercise. However, a word of caution: if using oxygen, do not use an electrically operated concentrator while in the pool. A small portable tank can be secured to pole or chair, and a 50' cannula used. Also, while in the pool, stay in water no deeper than mid-chest deep. If it's deeper, the weight of the water will act to compress the chest's expansion while you are breathing. So if restriction is felt, back up.

After a few weeks, there should be some progress and it's becoming apparent that improvements are possible. The initial kinks have been worked out and it's time to step it up a notch. How does one know when enough is enough, and when is it safe to progress? Remember the aerobic threshold point discussed earlier? The goal should be to achieve and sustain exercise between 60% and 80% of the aerobic threshold for about 30 to 50 cumulative minutes per session.

Determining that point is important and there are several methods that can be used. One is very scientific and several others are simple and easy to use: The **V-MaxO2** stress test will accurately identify your aerobic threshold and reference it to measurable values such as heart rate

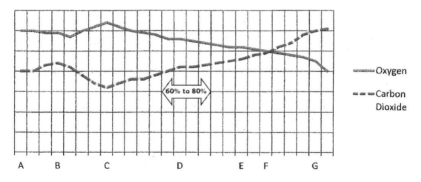

Exercise range defined.

or breathing that can then be easily monitored. This is very expensive and not very useful except for high-level athletes, so let's leave that one alone. If one is exercising at a fitness center, a trainer will probably calculate one's **target heart rate** and set a range to monitor. However, with a preexisting heart or lung problem, this calculation could be misleading. Nevertheless, since this calculation is commonly used in most fitness centers, it is important to be able to determine if this is a measurement that will be safe to use. The target heart rate is based on the maximum number of times (in theory, anyway) that the human heart is capable of beating in one minute. That number is 220 beats per minute for men as well as women. It's also assumed that this maximum decreases as we age (beginning to see the problem here?). So, subtracting your age from 220 will estimate the **maximum heart rate**. In theory, aerobic threshold should occur at the maximum heart rate. Optimal exercise should be between 60 to 80% of this target. For example:

75 years old: 75/yrs − 220/min. = 145/min.; 60% of 145 = 87/min. and 80% = 116/min.

If this person keeps their heart rate between 87 and 116, they should be getting enough of a workout, but not overdoing it. That's how it's supposed to work. However, remember that some pulmonary medicines may accelerate the heart rate, while some cardiac medicines may actually slow the heart rate. Therefore, relying totally on this estimation may not only be misleading but could be dangerous as well.

In a fitness center most likely there will be a chart on the wall called the **Borg Scale of Perceived Exertion**. This is an excellent tool to use, since it's you that's making the estimate as to how much effort is being put forth. There are many versions of this chart with more expanded scales, but using the scale of 1 to 10, try to stay in the 4–5 range during the first week of a new program. After a few weeks, progress exercise up to the 5–7 range as tolerated. Avoid progressing to levels 8 or 9; leave that to the young jocks. And 10—don't go there. The last thing one needs to do is get dizzy and fall off the treadmill. Another preferred method is tried and true: If while exercising, one can carry on a normal conversation without getting out of breath, it's unlikely that 80% of the maximum heart rate is being reached.

After a month or so, it's time to look back at the goals that were set at the beginning of the exercise program. Is sufficient progress being made or have the goals been achieved? If not, now is the time to reassess and adjust the routine. If using a home exercise program perhaps this would be a good time to review the current progress with the doctor. They may now recommend a professional at a fitness center, physical therapist or, better yet, a pulmonary rehabilitation program. If, however, there is satisfaction with the progress, now is not the time to quit but rather to move on to maintenance. Don't forget how much work it was to get back in shape, and remember that it only takes a few weeks of inactivity to slide back down. So don't stop.

The **maintenance routine** is slightly different from the initial investment. Most experts recommend aerobic exercise should be at least 30 minutes a day, *most* days of the week. For some with a busy schedule, that could be a problem. A problem perhaps, but not an excuse to quit. Actually, the good news is that breaking that half-hour up into two 15 minute or even three 10-minute

Perceived Exertion Scale
10 Have to stop NOW
9. Breathing VERY hard, legs giving out
8. Not much longer now; Gasping
7. Breathing hard, legs tired
6. I can still talk but getting it's harder
5. Breathing more noticeable
4. Starting to notice it now
3. Still comfortable. Breathing & legs OK
2. Piece of cake
1. I could do this all day

Perceived exertion scale.

sessions throughout the day will work as well as pounding it out for 30 minutes in a row. Many find that periodically alternating the schedule from time to time is a good way to keep it interesting.

One of the major excuses for stopping an exercise routine is that it becomes routine. "It's getting boring...." If so, a solution for this is **interval training**. Essentially, vary the exercise routine a bit. If walking is the primary exercise, try taking a different direction while walking around the block, or walk in a different neighborhood or a park. If using exercise equipment, try using different speeds, resistances or elevations for brief periods during each session. Interval training is very much like real life. If training on a treadmill at 2 mph at level grade, that's all well and good. However, in real life, while one is walking across the street to the donut shop and, halfway across, the light changes, that

2 mph on level ground isn't going to cut it. Real life situations occur all the time. Now with an improved level of conditioning, the addition of interval training prepares one for what the world is likely to dish out from time to time.

III. Strength Training: After a month or so, once aerobic condition has improved, consider strength training. Strengthening exercises help muscle fibers so that they are able to contract and work easier with less chance of injury. Don't expect to resemble somebody on muscle beach; that won't happen. Strength training will improve muscle tone, which is a state of partial contraction at rest. Muscles are used in conjunction with one another. For example, when bending an arm, muscles on one side have to shorten while the opposite side has to stretch. It takes energy to move those muscle fibers, and the farther they have to move, the more energy is required. If muscles are better toned, the same amount of work can be done with much less energy expenditure.

Strength training should not be done in lieu of aerobic conditioning; one does not replace the other. It is, however, fine to do strength training during the same sessions you do aerobics. Many find it better to alternate strength, then aerobics back and forth during each session. Although maintenance aerobics are recommended most days of the week, strength training should be no more than several times per week. It's recommended to allow at least one day off between strength training secessions. This will give the muscle fibers a chance to recover and lessen the chance of soreness or injury.

Begin strength training with a weight that's easy to move, not something that has to be struggled with. Strength training is measured in **repetitions (reps)** and **sets**. The rep is one complete (up and down or forward and back) cycle and a set is the number of repetitions completed before stopping to rest. Slowly inhale as the lift is begun and exhale while slowly returning the weight to rest. But don't let the weight come to a complete rest, keep it just a few inches from its stop in order to maintain tension to the muscles being used. The number of reps should be about 8–12 but limit the number of sets to 2 or 3. That will be enough to help develop strength without overdoing it. Never lift weights to the point of fatigue or when beginning to struggle. Doing so will only cause soreness and injury. Between sets, stop and rest for several minutes before attempting the next set, then reassess the level of fatigue. It's normal to become a little tired during the last several reps but not to feel significant discomfort. When a particular weight becomes *too* easy, increase the weight lifted with five-pound increments rather than increasing the reps or sets.

There are four basic strengthening techniques: free weights, machine weights, progressive resistance and isometrics. Each has its advantages and disadvantages, but the selection will more likely be based on availability than anything else.

Free weights: These are the classic dumbbells, but anything that has weight will work just as well. A 20 pound sack of potatoes or 1 pound bag of sugar will work just as well as store-bought weights. The use of free weights will most likely be hand weights that concentrate on arm and shoulder muscles. The advantage of free weights is there's no excuse because one can't find something to lift. Free weights can be used at home without the additional cost of going to a fitness center. They tend to develop a deeper level of muscle fiber intensity, since more muscles are used to maintain balance while one is lifting. These individual weights require an initial "dead weight" lift, which is the primary reason that the weight should not be excessive. Always take it slow and don't overdo it.

When lifting with the arms, the chest will always be involved. Be very careful of breath holding while lifting any weight. Inhale while lifting and exhale while lowering the weight. *Never, ever hold the breath while lifting a weight.* Breath holding while straining to lift a weight, increases the pressure in the chest, decreasing the pumping ability of the heart. This is known as the **Valsalva maneuver** and is dangerous; instead, breathe through the lift. If it feels necessary to hold the breath while lifting, the weight is too heavy. Don't lift it.

Machine weights: These are the machines likely to be found in a fitness center, although they are becoming popular in homes as well. The primary difference from a free weight is they tend to isolate the muscle group that is being used, which reduces the risk of inadvertent injury. Safety is always a concern while exercising and machine weights are ideal for beginners. The smoother movement lessens the chance of injury from overextending a muscle group or joint. Many seasoned high-level athletes also prefer these same machines for specific muscle training. Usually, in a fitness center, trainers are available to help properly adjust the equipment for optimal benefit.

Progressive resistance: These are the rubber bands or elastic tubes that are often used in rehabilitation centers. Unlike free weights, they don't rely on gravity to provide resistance. As the range of motion increases, so does the resistance, allowing for a smoother and therefore safer exercise. Minor changes in the angle allow for adjacent muscles to also be used which more accurately mimics movements during normal activities of daily living tasks. The advantage is that they are relatively inexpensive, lightweight and easily stored. They can be used with any muscle group so their versatility is limited only by one's imagination.

The only disadvantage is that both ends *must* be held, otherwise somebody is going to get snapped.

Isometrics: These strength exercises requires absolutely no equipment and can be done virtually anywhere. Contracting a particular muscle or group of muscles and holding that contraction is all that's required. This could also be accomplished by pushing against an immovable object such as a wall. Isometrics may be useful when particular joint limitations such as arthritis are involved since the muscle doesn't change length and the joint doesn't move. Isometrics aren't as efficient at increasing strength as other modalities but they are helpful in maintaining muscle tone in particular muscle sets. A repetition of 6 to 8 seconds followed with a brief rest of 10–15 seconds for 5–10 sets is sufficient. Advantages are that no equipment is required and they can be done anywhere, anytime. The disadvantage is they aren't intended to replace strength training, only supplement it. A word of caution, though: prolonged holding of a contraction can dramatically and quickly increase blood pressure. If cardiovascular problems such as hypertension, are part of one's medical history, keep the repetitions to a shorter duration.

IV. Recovery: Following each exercise session, it's time to cool down. Warming up and stretching out before exercising lessen the chance of injury during the session, while a proper cooldown helps keep muscles from becoming sore. Take at least five minutes to re-stretch those same muscles that were stretched during the initial warm-up.

Staying motivated: After a few months of aerobic and strength training some improvements should be obvious. Aerobic conditioning makes it easier to walk from the car to the house, while strength training makes it possible to also carry the groceries in from the car. It's just as important to continue an exercise program as it was to start one in the first place. It doesn't do much good to get into shape only to relapse to the same condition before all that hard work was done. In fact, research has shown that bouncing back and forth between fit and unfit can actually do more harm than good. The idea is to get fit and stay fit. Now is the time to develop a plan to maintain the level of conditioning that has been reached. A plan doesn't necessarily guarantee success, but without a plan, there's nothing to modify if needed. Here are some ideas to help:

1. Optimize breathing prior to an exercise routine. If necessary, use the prescribed rescue inhaler before having to stop and use it. "An ounce of prevention is worth a pound of cure."
2. If chronic pain such as arthritis limits flexibility, take any

recommended pain management medicine in sufficient time prior to exercising so the pain won't limit activities. If joint pain is a problem, take extra time to slowly stretch and warm up.

3. If oxygen is prescribed, during exercise it may be necessary to increase the flow from pulsed to continuous or increase the flow rate. But first *check with the doctor about doing so.* If the flow is increased during exercise, it's extremely important to return the flow to its normal rate when finished.

4. For obvious reasons, never exercise on a full stomach.

5. Make a pro/con list of the reasons for staying in shape. Feeling better as well as reducing medical expenses should be enough to motivate anyone.

6. Set realistic goals and keep a scorecard to review progress.

7. Lose the scale. Losing unwanted fat as a result of working out may be a good thing, but improving one's breathing and overall cardiopulmonary fitness is the primary objective.

8. Don't compare your progress to that of others. Everyone has their own goals, some of which may be different from yours. There will always be those who progress more rapidly than others. Everyone is different and will proceed at their own different rate. Don't be discouraged.

9. Work out with a buddy. Find someone that can help you maintain motivation and avoid discouragement. Carrying on a conversation while exercising will help monitor the end point of exertion.

10. Mix things up once in a while. Interval training adds variety and helps motivation.

11. Share those stated goals and your accomplishments with family and friends. If others know what you are trying to accomplish, their support will likely be encouraging.

12. Exercise doesn't always have to occur in a gym. Bowling and dancing are good aerobic activities where one can have fun while staying fit. Tai chi programs are excellent for improving flexibility, proper breathing control and stress management, so use them as well.

13. Reward yourself periodically. We all like to see some practical prize for our accomplishments. Go to the movies or out for a special dinner. Get a new exercise outfit and pat yourself on the back.

14. There will always be those days when you're not feeling well. It's important to watch for those warning signs and obey your body's needs. If it's time to stop and rest, do it. Conserve your strength for getting better.

Even with the best plan and faithfully following all the doctor's orders and suggestions, there will always be those episodes when illness will prevail. A trip to the emergency room or even a hospitalization. Scary times. But being more aware of the process may help reduce some of this anxiety. Let's turn to the next chapter for a behind the scenes look at what goes on.

Additional Reading

Duke Reeves, 28 February 2018, "How to Effectively Exercise at Home with COPD," // blog.lptmedical.com.
Joanna Soh, 30 April 2018, "How to Perform Proper Warm-up and Cool-Down Exercise," bing.com/videos.
"Exercises for Someone with COPD," www.copdfoundation.org.

12

Why Are They Doing Those Awful Things to Me in ICU?

Hopefully by now you have a better understanding of what's going on with breathing. Although the doctor is always the point person, there's a whole team of nurses, pharmacists, dietitians, case managers, and physical, occupational and respiratory therapists, all with specific roles to play in providing care. Even though a lot of resources are available, the most important link in this chain is *you*. If prescriptions aren't filled, or used correctly; if dietary recommendations aren't followed; if breathing techniques aren't used; if exercise regimens are ignored, there simply isn't much use in complaining that things aren't getting any better. Hopefully, the preceding chapters have shed some light on what the people in those various specialties are trying to do. Collaborative conversations are always more productive.

One needs to do a little more to prepare for an office visit than just show up on time. It's important to keep a list of concerns or questions to be asked. That way, when the doctor asks, "How you doing?" the conversation is more likely to be productive. It may seem like there's always another test that needs to be done. An important question seldom asked: "Are all those tests necessary?"

Obviously, the doctor has a reason for ordering those tests. Some are critical, while others help gauge progress and make sure medical management is on the right course. It's okay to ask about these tests; in fact most doctors are pleased that you're interested enough to ask. The doctor has an obligation to explain the purpose of those tests and procedures in terms that are able to be understood. This includes any potential risks and benefits as well as any alternatives that might be available. A legal form called **informed consent** is something which you will be asked to sign before anything (excluding emergency treatment) can be started. If there are any questions, have them answered. If unsure what was said, ask for someone else to explain it in terms that are able to be understood. It's that important. A few examples illustrate this.

Another one of our patients had a bad heart as well as bad lungs. In fact, she didn't have too much that was working well anymore. Cardiac catheterizations had been performed every year for the last five years and her doctor told her it was time for another one. She asked him simply, "If the results are better, will you take me off any of my medicine?" To which her doctor replied, "No, we can't reduce your medicines; you'll die." "Well then," she asked, "if the test is worse can you do surgery or add more medicines?" Again, her doctor replied, "No, you wouldn't survive surgery, and there aren't any more medicines I can offer; you're on everything there is." Her next question: "Then why are we doing it?" Her doctor agreed and the procedure was cancelled.

Because of emphysema, one of our elderly patients had been having annual pulmonary functions done at his local hospital. The results had always been dismal at best. Those of his latest one, a few months ago, were again clinically unchanged. He was surprised when his doctor called him to schedule another one in his office. It was explained that the doctor had recently purchased equipment so testing could now be conveniently done in the office rather than at the hospital and "baseline" studies needed to be done. He went and again the results were unchanged. A few months later, however, he was shocked to see that his insurance carrier would not pay for the additional testing, since it had been less than one year since his last pulmonary function. He was on the hook for the whole cost. Deductibles and co-pays can add up fast. Prior to an elective test always ask the office staff to check the insurer's coverage. True emergency testing and procedures are usually covered but non-emergency testing can be a different matter. Don't let the office staff get away with "We'll let you know what your insurance says after the test is done." A little late then.

However, even with the best of care, trips to the emergency department and occasionally hospitalizations will be needed. Scary as this may be, it's helpful to have a better understanding of what's going on. Let's take a brief look at what's going on behind the scenes.

In any size hospital, the emergency department can be a site of measured pandemonium. It takes a dedicated medical team to deal with everything that happens here. Life and death situations, to mumps and runny noses as well as the usual suspects just looking for a place to spend the night. The team's range of skills is constantly being tested, from tending to the needs of newborn babies to those of the very elderly.

Emergency departments don't treat patients on a first-come, first-serve basis. That's why they have a **triage nurse** do a quick assessment. The most unstable patients will be seen by the doctor first. Unless it's a life or death emergency, the triage nurse will be the first stop for one when arriving in the emergency department. One's current symptoms will be evaluated and vital signs measured. The results will determine how quickly one needs to be seen by the doctor. Don't be fooled by those popular billboards advertising up-to-the-minute wait times. What they are showing is how long it may take to get registered and see the triage nurse, not necessarily the doctor. Questions will be asked about symptoms and how long they have been bothersome, current medicines and when they were last taken. Be prepared for these questions; they help the triage nurse more accurately assess what's needed. Above all else, be patient; you don't know what else is going on back there.

More questions again! Doctors, nurses, therapists, radiology technicians are all asking things that they need to know. What's not of particular importance to one specialist may be important to another. For example, the question of pregnancy might not be of particular interest to the respiratory therapist, but would be for the radiologist. So be patient. Depending on your condition, an intravenous line (IV) may be inserted in one's hand or arm, even if one was put in by the paramedics in the ambulance. They had selected a larger vein that was quick to get to but not necessarily suited for longer-term use. Be patient, don't object. The nurses know what's needed and, no, they aren't just poking holes because they enjoy it. Blood samples can often be drawn from the IV, saving one a lot of discomfort. Additionally, medicine can be administered directly into the IV for faster results. More importantly, if for any reason there should be a sudden drop in blood pressure, finding a suitable vein will be much more difficult. It's important to have a good working line as soon as possible.

By now the doctor has been in and x-ray and lab tests have been completed. All results are evaluated quickly but sometimes they indicate that additional testing is needed. The tests ordered will be determined by the current symptoms. Some may take a little longer to complete, while others may require serial samples a few hours apart. Although similar tests may have been recently done in the doctor's office, the emergency department doctor needs to know what's going on right now, so don't object. If breathing is the problem, oxygen will likely be administered in sufficient doses to raise the blood oxygen to safer levels. Additional breathing treatments will likely be given even though they may have recently been taken at home. Arterial blood gases may be tested to assess the ability of the lungs to carry oxygen and exhale carbon dioxide.

Even though these tests and procedures will likely be started and completed quickly, the attending doctor needs to see if "the fix sticks." Nothing is accomplished if one leaves in 20 minutes feeling better but has to make a U-turn in the parking lot and come back.

Hopefully by now things should have gotten a little better, or at least been stabilized for the moment. The doctor now needs to decide what to do next. The process goes something like this: Are you well enough to go home and, if so, competent enough to take care of yourself? If so, you'll probably be discharged home with instructions to follow up with your **primary care doctor**. If help will be needed at home, is there someone who is capable of helping (and willing)? Unless the answer is anything but a resounding yes, they need to find you a place that is able to administer the proper level of care. If conditions warrant, placement in the hospital's **acute care** will be made. Nurses will administer care under the direction of either your **primary care doctor** or a **hospitalist** whose medical practice is limited to hospitalized patients. If a higher or specialized level of care is needed, admission to an **intensive care unit (ICU)** will be arranged. In larger hospitals, there may be numerous ICUs specializing in medical, surgical, coronary, neurological as well as several other focused care disciplines. The availability of these specialized services is limited.

Admission to the ICU can be a scary time for you as well as any family members. Monitoring electrodes and IVs may have to be changed again to accommodate more advanced devices. More questions again for the same varied reasons as in the emergency department. Be patient. It isn't because the staff isn't communicating; they just need to make sure nothing has been missed. Alarms and beeps will be a constant in the ICU. These are the sounds that the nurses and therapists are listening to all the time. Although not every sound or alarm will bring a host of people running, the staff are well trained to distinguish the difference between those sounds. The alarm thresholds are usually set rather tight so if a parameter limit is exceeded, a responding alarm will result. Even though someone isn't always physically present in the room, someone is always watching at a remote monitor and will send help immediately if needed. Just be patient.

The number of IVs hanging on the pole is not an indication of the severity of one's illness. Don't count the bags and get worried. Tubes may need to be inserted in the mouth, nose, bladder, rectum, veins, arteries and just about any other place that God never intended for tubes to go. They are there for a reason. Restraints may be needed to keep those lines and tubes from accidentally being pulled out. Remember what it's like at home when waking up after a deep sleep and being momentarily confused? That happens a lot in ICU. It isn't fun to be tied down, but if it's necessary, it's for one's own good. So be patient. ICU is an around-the-clock job. Activity doesn't slow down at night, and when one is sleeping on and off all day and night it's easy to get a little mixed up. Don't fight with the nurses; they're trying to help. Disorientation is not an uncommon side effect of spending a few days in an intensive care unit. Higher doses of sedation and other medications often result in confusion. Things will straighten out once you are stabilized. Be patient.

Different types of oxygen equipment may be needed depending on prevailing circumstances. Pressure ventilation with a CPAP (continuous positive airway pressure) or BiPAP (bilevel positive airway pressure) may temporarily be used. They can give the overworked breathing muscles a rest while other medications have a chance to work. The terms **ventilator** and **respirator**, often used interchangeably, refer to life support equipment. A tube will need to be placed in the lungs (**intubation**) so that ventilation can be adjusted and closely monitored. The tube is placed between the vocal cords, so talking won't be possible until the tube has been removed (**extubated**). Although ventilators are used as life support measures, they are by no means the last resort. Continuous monitoring by doctors, nurses and respiratory therapists will be able to determine when it's safe to resume normal (**spontaneous**) breathing.

When in the hospital, one of the most frequent complaints is that the doctor only looked in the door, mumbled, "How are you today?" and then left. However, before coming to the room, they have already reviewed test results as well as nursing notes. In other words, when they ask how you're doing—they already know. Nevertheless, they are there to answer any questions. If they say that you're not yet ready to go home, it's fair to ask why. Don't be in a big rush to go home. There were reasons for the hospital admission, and the last thing anyone wants is for you to go home too soon and return that night because of the same thing.

Alternative care comes into play when one is not sick enough to remain in the hospital but not well enough to care for oneself at home. A **visiting nurse** or **skilled nursing assistant** who comes to the home as necessary to check one's progress may be all that's needed. If closer supervision is needed, **sub-acute or rehabilitation facilities** are designed for those who can basically perform some but not all of their own self-care. These are not long-term facilities but rather are designed to help one make a smoother and safer transition to home.

Sometimes, however, going home with a return to independent living are no longer options in the foreseeable future. In that case, there are other options available and the doctor will have a **case manager** assist with making those decisions and arrangements. **Assisted**

living facilities are designed for those who may not be candidates for returning to independent living but are still able to provide the majority of their personal care. They can offer a higher level of assistance with non-medical activities of daily living such as dressing, bathing and toileting. Once the doctor has determined the level of care that is needed following discharge, the case manager will compile a list of facilities that will accept your insurance and have openings for new residents. If possible, visit the facility or have a family member or friend visit to get an overview of what conditions are like before accepting placement.

For those who don't qualify for assisted living options and the sub-acute or rehabilitation placement is no longer optional, then it may be time to consider a **nursing home**. As compared to residents of assisted living facilities, residents of nursing homes generally require more support with activities of daily living and sometimes total care. As providers of long-term care, nursing home are subject to frequent inspections to ensure residents receive a high quality of care in a well-maintained setting. Although not all nursing home residents will be be as active as their counterparts, an **activities director** organizes activities that encourage socializing and promote well-being.

Hospice is a type of care and philosophy that focuses on the palliative care of the chronically or terminally ill to relieve pain and symptoms. Additionally, hospices also focus on the family's individual emotional and spiritual needs. Hospice care is not a reduction or lower level of medical care. It's a level of care that focuses on quality of life instead of on continuing with curative treatment simply to prolong life. Patients qualifying for hospice care may receive services as an inpatient in an assisted living facility or nursing home. However, **hospice at home** may also be available for those who wish to remain in the familiar surroundings of home. Under hospice care, basic medical care is continued with a focus on pain and symptom control. Medical supplies and needed equipment are provided and team members are available 24/7 as needed. Respite care is available for family and others who regularly provide daily care but may need a break from time to time. Volunteer support for tasks such as preparing meals and running errands is also available as needed. Assisting with end of life arrangements and continued counseling and supportive care for the loved one's family, once the loved one has passed away, is also an essential priority of hospice philosophy.

Whew, that last part was kind of a downer, wasn't it? However, life has a beginning as well as an end. It's all connected, and although we don't like to dwell on it, the importance of making final plans can't be emphasized enough. None of us wants to sit around thinking about what "could happen" should our ability to make our wishes known be lost. However, a little planning now is much better than handing those decisions down to family members who will forever carry the burden of wondering if they made the "right" decision. Unfortunately, when multiple family members have to make those decisions, differences of opinion can pull families apart at a time when they need to be drawn together. The worst-case scenario is for those decisions to finally be made in a court of law by people who know nothing about you.

There are two basic documents for making one's wishes known. The first is a **living will**, which describes the limits to the level of care one wishes to have. This document should not be confused with a conventional will, which is designed for leaving property after death. A common misconception is that once a living will is signed, it can't be changed. But it *can* be changed and often is. Even with a living will your wishes will supersede any previous declarations made in a living will. It is intended to let your wishes be known if (for lack of a better term) heroic, life-sustaining measures are needed and you aren't able to communicate an informed decision.

The aspect most people associate with living wills is the **do not resuscitate (DNR)** order. What is not well understood are the various degrees of resuscitation available. If the heart stops beating adequately, sometimes all it takes for a person to be revived are basic **advanced cardiac life support (ACLS)** drugs. It may be possible to support breathing with a CPAP or BiPAP, avoiding intubation and mechanical ventilation. These measures may only be needed on a temporary basis until you are stabilized. Other aspects of the living will could stipulate the desire for renal dialysis or a feeding tube placement which may be required for prolonged use to sustain life.

The second document often used, along with a living will, is a **durable power of attorney**. This will be someone, named by you, to make any additional health care decisions that you may not have otherwise expressed. A designated power of attorney is recommended in the event that additional decisions regarding care need to be made that may not have been known at the time the living will went into effect. These documents do not imply a reduced level of care. Taking just a few minutes to prepare these documents is not "throwing in the towel" by any means. It's simply making your wishes known, so loved ones are reassured that the right choices will be made when needed.

Of course, an *extended* trip to the emergency department or even a *brief* hospitalization can be a frightening experience at best. However, aren't you glad the resources are there when needed? It might seem that these trips are occurring all too often. In the next chapter, let's look at a few other conditions besides asthma or COPD that can also compromise breathing and sometimes result in those frantic trips for emergency treatment.

Additional Reading

Maureen Welker, MSN, NP, CCRN, 22 June 2017, "ICU (Intensive Care Unit): Tips for Patients and Families," www.onhealth.com.
Lisa Esposito, 20 November 2016, "What to Expect When Your Loved One Is in the ICU," www.health.usnews.com.
Lisa Esposito, 12 June 2014, "Your Rights as a Hospital Patient," www.health.usnews.com.

13

What About
Other Common
Breathing Problems?

Since breathing occupies the better part of our lives, even minor complications are noticeable. Unfortunately, with chronic lung disease already slowing things down, those minor sniffles become more than just a nuance. The coughing, wheezing and shortness of breath are now a big deal. Unfortunately, a preexisting lung disease doesn't give one a free pass with the ordinary maladies that most everyone encounters. In fact, the risk of catching what "goes around" is now even greater. Let's examine a few of those problems that occur from time to time, and look for precautions that can be taken.

Germs

Basically, there are four kinds of microorganisms capable of making us sick: bacteria, viruses, fungi and protozoa. They are found everywhere and are quite adaptable to ever-changing situations. The reality is that these microorganisms don't live in our world; we live in theirs. Not all of them are bad; in fact, many are beneficial and essential for our health and the well-being of the environment. Normally, we get along well together—as long as they stay where they belong. Unfortunately, not all are helpful, and when these organisms result in disease they are collectively referred to as **germs**.

Fungi normally are spore-producing microorganisms. They aren't members of the plant or animal kingdom, and in fact are their own kingdom. They live in moist environments and are beneficial in breaking down and recycling decaying organisms to enrich the soil. If we enjoy mushrooms on our pizza or have ever used penicillin to get better, thank a fungus.

A fungus infection, however, is difficult to treat. If a damaged roof or leaking pipe causes moisture to accumulate in a wall, mold is likely to develop. Spores are then released and find their way into circulating air. Asthmatic attacks can be severe and prolonged as long as the mold is not removed.

Normally, our mouths contain numerous organisms. As long as their individual population remains normal, they all get along fine. When using a steroidal inhaler an overgrowth of **yeasts** can occur in some (not all) patients, resulting in a severe sore throat known as **thrush** (as discussed in Chapter 3). This isn't something that is caught from the inhaler. Steroids tend to dampen down the immune system and, in some people, this can cause a yeast overgrowth. It is strongly recommended that after using a steroidal inhaler one vigorously rinse the mouth with water in order to reduce the risk of thrush.

Protozoa are single-celled organisms that are also widely found in nature. They prefer water or other moist environments. They help enrich the soil and normally are not much of a problem unless one consumes contaminated water or food.

Bacteria, on the other hand, are the most abundant life-form on the planet. They have adapted to live in even the most inhospitable environments. Bacteria are essential in the digestion of our food, among other things. Unfortunately, not all bacteria are helpful, and those that can cause disease such TB, pneumonia, and tetanus can be deadly. *Pseudomonas* is a common bacterium found virtually everywhere. It needs moisture to survive, which is a particular concern for anyone using nebulizers or humidifiers, where moisture may remain following use. The importance of regularly cleaning inhalation equipment cannot be stressed enough. Since bacteria are living organisms, they can be destroyed by our immune system but sometimes one needs a little help with the proper antibiotic.

Viruses are not considered living organisms. Actually, a virus is a bridge between the living and non-living. They are so small that hundreds of viruses could fit on one bacteria. Unlike living cells, a virus cannot consume food or excrete waste. Nor can it grow, reproduce or migrate on its own. It consists of a tiny bit of genetic material that is wrapped in a protective coat for protection. Its existence depends on attaching to a host cell and injecting its genetic material. It then uses the host's reproductive mechanisms to make more little viruses. The host cell eventually dies, ruptures and releases more viruses to repeat the process. In order to be successful, a virus needs to be passed to another host. This typically occurs from direct transmission via a careless sneeze or cough. Millions of aerosolized viruses are able to be briefly suspended in the air, which can then be inhaled by anyone in close proximity. Viruses can also survive on some surfaces for a short while. Transmission then becomes possible when that surface is touched and the virus is manually transferred to the new host's eyes, nose or mouth.

The common cold, or **upper respiratory infection** (URI), is caused by viruses which are normally present all year. More often than not, our immune system is able to keep them in check and we aren't even aware of the occasional thwarted attack. However, certain times of the year the viruses are more prevalent and easily transmitted. During seasonal changes, our body is going through a recalibration of sorts. Although one may be looking forward to the change, the disruption in daily rhythms often keeps the immune system from doing its job properly. Disruption of sleep cycles, and changing weather patterns may increase stress levels, increasing vulnerability. Holiday festivities often bring people in closer quarters where even one careless sneeze can disperse millions of viruses. By the way, a URI can't be caught unless one comes in contact with the virus. Going outside with wet hair, not eating enough veggies or not getting enough sleep won't result in a cold. Nevertheless, those things do detract from the immune system's ability to do its job—which is protecting you, so be careful.

The virus typically enters the respiratory track via the nose or mouth and symptoms usually begin there. Onset is usually slow during the first several days, while the virus is busy making more little viruses. Other than mild chills (which is where the cold got its name) other symptoms may not yet be apparent. Unfortunately, during these first few days, lesser amounts of the virus can still be spread to others. Around the third day or so, enough virus has been produced that additional symptoms are becoming noticeable. A sore or scratchy throat, stuffy or runny nose with sneezing or coughing. During this time, spreading the virus to others is more likely due to the increased number of viruses now present. The cold virus is usually self-limiting and symptoms gradually subside in about a week or so. Treating the symptoms won't necessarily speed the healing process but will make one feel better. And minimizing those uncomfortable symptoms will reduce stress and help one get the rest that is needed so the immune system can do its job.

More often than not, Mom's advice to drink plenty of fluids and get extra rest will be sufficient. Of course, common sense needs to prevail and one should consult the doctor if there are any questions. A sore throat may be relieved by gargling with warm salt water several times per day and especially at night. Aspirin or similar products can be used as necessary to relieve mild fever and reduce body aches. An over-the-counter antihistamine and/or expectorant may help relieve a stuffy or runny nose and a cough. However, make sure the cough isn't the result of asthmatic symptoms, which may trigger bronchospasms. If bronchodilators are prescribed for as needed use, they should be used as a prophylaxis rather than waiting for breathing to get worse. It's unclear if the use of zinc lozenges or increased dosages of vitamin C actually prevents or reduces the length of a URI. There is, however, some evidence that they may lessen symptoms. In view of the fact that the use of zinc is capable of producing undesirable side effects, it's best to consult the doctor.

There are well over 200 viruses that are responsible for the common cold, any one of which could result in a URI. It seems strange that in this era of modern medicine there isn't a cure or vaccine for the common cold. Unfortunately, a virus is not alive so it can't be killed and a vaccine to cover all potential varieties is not practicable. When symptoms are first noticed, several days have already passed. A culture would then be needed to determine which variety of virus was present and which vaccine to use. Then after waiting a few days for the results to come back, the effects of the virus would about be over anyway. The old saying seems to hold some truths: Treat a cold aggressively and it will be gone in about seven days, but if left to run its course, it takes about a week.

Influenza is also a virus but the symptoms tend to be a little worse than those of the common cold. As opposed to a cold, influenza symptoms usually develop rapidly. A higher fever often accompanied with a headache and lower back ache and just "feeling bad all over" are more typical of influenza. The symptoms are usually self-limiting and gradually improve in seven to ten days. Symptoms of nausea, vomiting and diarrhea are actually related to **gastroenteritis,** or inflammation of the lining of the stomach or intestines. Vomiting and diarrhea are the most prevalent symptoms and usually only last several (long) days. Gastroenteritis is caused by either **norovirus** or bacterial infection, whereas the influenza virus is a respiratory event.

It's important to note that complications are more common with influenza as opposed to with URIs. Preexisting chronic medical problems predispose one to secondary infections while the influenza is running its course. Therefore, Mom's advice may need to be amended a little bit, and one should consult the doctor, who may order a course of antibiotics to prevent secondary infections from occurring. And when antibiotics are prescribed, be sure to take them as directed. Using them for just a "few days," until feeling better, is inviting a disaster. If those germs are knocked down but not out, it leaves them a chance to regroup and develop a resistance to that particular antibiotic. In medical slang, they are now known as a **super bug** and can be really hard to knock out the second time around.

Unlike the common cold, there are only four varieties of the influenza virus. As mutations occur, various sub-types of that particular virus will develop. Of the four basic varieties, two may cause severe symptoms, one only mild symptoms and one only affects animals and birds. Prior to each flu season, scientists are able to determine which of the three varieties are likely to be making the rounds. A specific influenza type of vaccine is then developed and is normally available in early autumn. Although it won't necessarily prevent one from catching the flu bug, it significantly improves the odds against it. And if symptoms do develop, they tend to be less troublesome.

While the body is recovering from a bout of the flu, the immune system develops natural antibodies to protect against future exposures to that particular strain. Unfortunately, over time, small changes in the surface proteins of the virus may undergo an **antigenic drift**. Fortunately, these small changes remain closely related to the original virus. As a result, antibodies developed as a result of a vaccine or recovering from that particular viral sub-type will still offer some **cross protection**. However, accumulated mutations over time may eventually cause significant changes to the point where the immune system may not be able to provide adequate protection. Therefore, re-infection is not necessarily a result of the vaccine or our immune system failing but rather a "reengineering" of the virus. The best advice is to get the flu shot early, since it takes several weeks for it to be most effective. If you are over the age of 65 or have chronic medical conditions, ask if a high-dose vaccine would be more appropriate. When it comes right down to it, *an ounce of prevention is worth a pound of cure.* So, let's talk about prevention.

Since airborne particles seem to be the most efficient way of spreading these germs, be courteous to others and cover your cough. Dispose of used tissues properly, and if caught unprepared for a sneeze, use the crook of the elbow rather than the hand. Protection from someone else's errant, unanticipated sneeze is often easier said than done. Droplets from a forceful sneeze or cough may spread a considerable distance. Keeping a reasonable **social distance** of about 6 feet or so helps reduce the likelihood of transmission. The operative word here is "reduce," since droplets will be affected by the forcefulness of a cough or sneeze as well as air currents. In a crowded room the chances of transmission are substantially increased.

Although a face mask is a good idea, it doesn't necessarily

guarantee protection. To be effective, it must be worn properly. To a certain extent, a facial mask will restrict breathing. As a result, many opt for wearing it only over their mouth while the nose is exposed. Since air is also entrained via the nose, airborne germs are carried along with the flow. The mask must be fitted snugly to reduce air entrainment around the edges of the mask. Between uses, storing of the mask in a plastic or paper bag is not advised. The outside of the mask must be considered contaminated while the inside (facing you) is considered clean. In a storage bag, cross contamination is more likely to occur. And of course, don't share used masks. Face shields are preferred by some; however, unless a mask is also worn, protection is limited. Inhaled air will be pulled from around the shield and unfiltered air subsequently inhaled.

Another mode of transmission is from hands to face. It's unlikely you can see what's on that doorknob or shared computer terminal. Using a handrail when walking up or down public stairs, one probably encounters enough germs to infect half the country. If a handrail is needed for stability, use the edge of the fist rather than the open hand. Even if contaminated, that part of the hand is less likely to come in contact with one's eyes, nose or mouth. And of course, the intimacy of the friendship hug or handshake should be avoided during those times when the cold and flu are more prevalent. They'll understand.

Most of us inadvertently touch our face, nose, mouth or eyes an average of 200 times each day and never even realize it. Therefore, the frequency and adequacy of handwashing are essential in reducing the transmission of germs. Soap and running water seem to be the active ingredient. Warm water is best but it's the running water that is the key. And don't just wash the fingertips, wash between the fingers and the back of the hands as well. How long to wash? Recommendations of 20 seconds, or about the length of time it takes to sing the "Happy Birthday" song, should be sufficient. And while already at the sink, consider washing your face. Airborne particles can land there as well. No need for a full scrub, but a gentle rinse, wiping outward away from the nose and mouth, may help.

Many feel that wearing gloves is adequate protection from germs. Just remember, though, that germs will get on the gloves just as easily as they get on the hands. And then if you touch your face, an infection can occur just as easily as if you had gone without gloves in the first place. Hand sanitizers help, but the majority are alcohol based, which can dry the skin. Dry, cracked skin is also a portal for infections. If using hand sanitizers frequently, be sure to occasionally use a moisturizer cream as well.

Hospital workers encounter germs all the time. That's just part of the job. To decrease the chance of acquiring or spreading germs, most have learned to use their non-dominant hand to turn knobs or in other everyday actions. Pushing open swinging doors with the upper arm or hip makes hand contamination less likely. If a door handle is all that's available for pulling open a door, use a tissue on the handle. If wearing long sleeves, pull a sleeve down a little to protect the hand. If nothing else, consider using the little finger of your non-dominant hand to open the door. Although this won't provide the needed protection, you are less likely to scratch the next facial itch with that little finger of your non-dominant hand.

Influenza Epidemic and Pandemics

By and large the *normal* seasonal influenza slows things down a bit. However, with a flu shot and a little extra vigilance, it's not a big deal. After all, when everyone's coughing and sneezing, a medical degree isn't needed to know that something's going around. Even at that, the distribution of germs is usually limited and not widely spread. A community outbreak such as this is known as an **epidemic**. Fortunately, the annual flu shot is about 70% effective in reducing the spread within the community. Unfortunately, not everyone is willing to take advantage of this protection, but enough do to slow the progression. Because of this, normal activities such as school and work are not seriously affected. Equally importantly, since the outbreak is somewhat limited, there is reduced strain on medical resources.

Viruses (as well as other germs) naturally mutate and select attributes that make them more successful. Rather than becoming more lethal, evolution usually moves in the direction of improving a virus's ability to reproduce. When the virus is able to mutate from an animal or bird population and acquires the ability to infect humans, the mutation may result in a major change of new surface proteins. The result is a new sub-type of influenza virus. This is known as an **antigenic shift**. Although rare, when it does occur, the outbreak quickly spreads and will now be termed a **pandemic**. When a new (**novel**) mutation is first introduced into a population, no one has yet had a chance to develop antibodies for protection. Vaccines for this new sub-type will have to be developed, produced and administered. As a result, there is an abrupt and near exponential increase in the rate of infections.

Pandemics seem to occur several times each century. The Spanish Influenza of 1918 claimed an estimated 100 million lives worldwide. Since then millions more have died as the result of the Asian flu (1957), the Hong Kong flu (1968) and more recently the 2003 SARS virus and the 2009 swine flu. Fortunately, medical science has learned much during these pandemics. Therapeutics as well as emphasis on personal hygiene have improved outcomes. As the infection quickly escalates, medical resources become overwhelmed. Additionally, because closer proximity increases the rate of transmission, the ability for people in affected locales to work and gather together must be limited. Essential services such as sanitation and health care are compromised, further compounding the strain on society as it tries to cope.

The most recent global pandemic involved COVID-19, the disease caused by the **SARS-CoV-2** virus. **Coronavirus** is a generic term that includes a large family of viruses named for the bulb-tipped spikes that project from the virus's surface. These spikes give it the appearance of a surrounding corona. As the name implies: SARS (Severe Acute Respiratory Syndrome), CO (corona family of viruses), VI (virus), D (disease), **19** (the year first identified). This newer virus is similar to the SARS-associated outbreak in 2003 and therefore is designated SARS-CoV-2. Unfortunately, this newest mutation has developed several modifications to aid its ability to infect and reproduce. Many otherwise healthy young adults are infected, but because their symptoms remain subclinical, they continue with work, school and social gathering. Unfortunately, the virus is then unknowingly transmitted to others who may be more susceptible.

Since viruses are typically spread by aerosolized particles, upper respiratory infections are where symptoms usually first occur. When first infected, our cells normally have antiviral alarms that send out a call for help. The SARS-CoV-2 virus is able to disrupt those signals, thus giving it additional time to reproduce before symptoms are first noticed.

For most viruses, the limiting factor in reproducing and surviving is the difficulty in attaching to a host's cell in order to deposit genetic material. The mutations of SARS-CoV-2 have overcome this problem. The virus is attracted to and sticks to a protein called ACE2 which is found on the outside of most cells. They are particularly abundant in the lungs, heart, blood vessels and kidneys. This virus is able to attach about 10 times easier and has a stronger connection than previous viruses. The viral spikes, necessary for transferring its genetic material, consist of two connected halves which must separate in order to enter the host cell. For most viruses, this separation isn't always successful. The SARS-CoV-2 mutation has found a way to use an enzyme normally produced by our cells to easily cut the spike so the genetic material can be successfully injected.

Due to the tight bonding and the virus's ability to inject its genetic material and replicate more viruses, a severe infection may be underway by the time the body's symptoms first appear. As a result, a severe pneumonia is more likely to become a major complication of this infection. Unfortunately, the virus doesn't stop there and may continue on and seek out additional ACE2 protein receptors and infect other organ systems like the heart, blood vessels and kidneys. In short, the SARS-CoV-2 virus is a lot more dangerous than just a seasonal flu.

Patients who are most seriously affected often have preexisting medical conditions of diabetes, obesity or hypertension. The common factor in these conditions is chronic inflammation. Infection with the SARS-CoV-2 virus results in the release of cytokines. These are chemical messengers that trigger inflammation in an effort to fight the infection. This is a normal and proper response to any infection. However, when chronic inflammation is already a factor, it can become overwhelming to the extent that non-infectious cells are also damaged and killed. This is referred to as a **cytokine storm**.

The ACE-2 protein plays a major role in regulating blood pressure. As a result, anyone with untreated hypertension is at a greater risk for complications. The excessive blood pressures and inflammation can destabilize and cause previously asymptomatic fatty plaque to be sheared free, resulting in emboli. Additionally, high fevers and low oxygen levels are irritating to the heart muscle and can lead to abnormal heart rhythms, further compromising recovery and survival. Fever and inflammation are also contributing factors to blood clot formations. Strokes and myocardial infarctions may result from these additional emboli. Micro clots may also lodge in the kidneys and lead to renal failure requiring dialysis or kidney transplant.

Any pandemic initially claim the lives of those whose immune systems are not fully developed or are weakened by age or preexisting medical conditions—the very young and old. Even though having preexisting lung disease may not necessarily cause one to be more susceptible to infection, when one's pulmonary reserves are already limited, any disruption is likely to become serious.

Although initial infection rates increase nearly exponentially, the rates gradually level off and decline. Even in this age of modern medicine, these pandemics normally persist about a year or so before they gradually dissipate. As the pandemic progresses and more people recover, natural antibodies are produced. This acquired immunity now provides protection that wasn't there before. With fewer people as active carriers, there will be fewer transmissions. As a result, the ability of that virus to persist will be limited. Vaccines that are ultimately produced will further decrease the likelihood of this particular mutation from returning, at least as a pandemic extreme.

Will there be pandemics in the future? If history is any indicator, of course there will. Will medical science provide solutions? Most likely, but as with any viral infection, prevention is the key. Unless the virus is transmitted to a new host, the protective protein coating of the virus will eventually fail and the virus will no longer be infectious. This protective coating is easily destroyed with soap and water, but such tools must be used to be effective. Face masks and social distancing to reduce the aerosolized exchange are also effective, but they can't be sporadically used. All it takes is one unprotected moment for one to become infected and continue the spread. While waiting for medical science to come to the rescue, these simple measures are the same ones that helped bring the 1918 pandemic to an end.

Allergies: Everyone is allergic to something. Most of us would react to poison ivy, but if we never encounter it we'll never have a problem. And that's the whole key to allergies—avoidance. Unfortunately, there are those things in the environment that are unavoidable. Pollens, molds, fumes and pet dander, just to name a few. These are called **allergens**, and if sensitive to them, the body will react with symptoms similar to those of a cold such as sneezing and coughing. Unlike with the common URI, though, red irritated eyes will be a more frequent symptom. The symptoms are the body's immune system trying to provide protection but making one miserable in the meantime. Unlike viral infections, allergic reactions don't run their course and go away. A doctor (**allergist**) may administer small injections of the allergens which, over a period of time, help decrease the intensity of symptoms. Over-the-counter remedies such as antihistamines are useful to relieve some symptoms.

The most common allergens are of the airborne variety, such as pollen, and when we're out and about, pollen that settles in our hair will fall onto the pillow at night. It's then likely to be inhaled, resulting in nighttime and early morning symptoms. Simply damp-rinsing one's hair before bed and/or changing the pillowcase before sleeping may be helpful in reducing the amount of pollen inhaled.

Seasonal allergies usually occur when various pollens are more prevalent. If so, work out a plan with the doctor to begin preventive measures such as using antihistamines, bronchodilators or eye drops several weeks prior to, during, and for several weeks after these seasonal events. The daily pollen counts in one's local area can be found in the daily paper or on the internet. If increased pollen counts are anticipated, rescheduling elective outdoor activities or taking appropriate precautions may minimize one's exposure.

Pneumonia is an accumulation of fluid in the alveoli of the lungs, the air-filled sacs that are the entry and exit point for gas exchange with the blood. In spite of the many advances in medicine, pneumonia still ranks as one of the leading causes of death. The fluid accumulation is usually due to an infection which also causes irritation and inflammation. The influenza virus is the most common cause of pneumonia. However, there are over 30 different causes, including bacteria, other viruses, fungus and even the aspiration of fluids or food. That upper respiratory infection that was ignored the last week or so may now have evolved into pneumonia.

Pneumonias are often described by their location as well as the causative agent. For example, **lobar pneumonia** is pneumonia confined to a section (lobe) of a lung.

Bronchial pneumonia results in multiple patches of infiltrates in one or both lungs.

Atypical pneumonia, often called **walking pneumonia**, is caused by a bacterium known as *Mycoplasma pneumoniae*. Although symptoms are normally mild, this condition can progress to severe if not treated. It's been said that men, rather than women, are more likely to contract walking pneumonia just because men can be too stubborn to go to the doctor. After walking around for a week or so they finally have no other choice.

Interstitial pneumonia is an unusual form of pneumonia that is characterized by persistent scarring of both lungs which may progress to pulmonary fibrosis. In reaction to a lung infection, the immune response is inflammation. Excessive and unimpeded inflammation is what leads to scarring. Although some autoimmune diseases may be contributory, the majority of cases are listed as **idiopathic**, or cause unknown.

Pneumococcal pneumonia is caused by the **streptococcus** bacterium and represents about 30% of diagnosed pneumonias. Fortunately, there is a vaccine available for this form of pneumonia. Although this vaccine won't protect one from every possible type of pneumonia, it does cover about 20 varieties that are caused by the streptococcus bacteria. Follow the doctor's advice and get the pneumonia shot if it's recommended.

Aspiration pneumonia isn't caused by an infection but rather foods or fluids that are partially inhaled into the lungs. Swallowing is actually a complicated maneuver we never even have to think about. If, however, there is a neurological problem, such as a stroke, the ability to protect the airway while swallowing could be compromised. In this case, pneumonia will usually be seen in the right lung, since this bronchus is more aligned with the trachea.

Hypostatic pneumonia ("hypo" = less than normal; "static" = little or no movement) is a collection of fluids (pooling) in the gravity-dependent (lower) portions of the lungs. It's most often the result of inactivity and more likely to affect the elderly or those who are confined to bed for a prolonged period of time due to illness or injury. Fluids in the body are affected by gravity and normally, when we're up and around, fluids keep circulating as they normally should. Unfortunately, even a few days of remaining in one position can result in a pooling of fluids, and in the lungs, that's pneumonia. That's why the nurses and respiratory therapists are constantly getting their patients out of bed or at least turning them from side to side every few hours.

With a preexisting chronic lung disease, development of a pneumonia can quickly evolve from minor distress to a critical situation. But how does one know when to call the doctor? Most often the advice is to monitor temperature, shortness of breath and coughing up mucus. Unfortunately, with COPD or asthma, two out of those three symptoms may be the norm. Therefore, evaluation of symptoms must always be calibrated to what is normal for *you*:

Symptoms: Normally, a URI or the flu will produce uncomfortable symptoms. They should, however, begin to dissipate after 3–5 days. If the intensity of symptoms worsens or they simply do not improve, call the doctor.

Temperature: If doing vital sign checks daily (as discussed in Chapter 9) an increase from what is normal *for you* should be evident. Moderate elevations above 100 degrees should prompt further investigation.

Amount and color of mucus: If the amount coughed up has increased or there is a significant color change, call the doctor. Pneumonia often increases the frequency and forcefulness of coughing. As a result, small streaks of blood may be seen in the mucus.

Shortness of breath: Because of chronic lung disease, dyspnea may be normal for you. If, however, your activity is now more limited and recovery is prolonged because of breathing or excessive fatigue, call the doctor.

Pleurisy is an inflammation of the **pleura**, the moist double-layered membranes that cover the lungs and line the inside of the chest wall. It is a very common condition and may accompany a bacterial or viral infection, such as an upper respiratory infection or the flu. It may, however, be present without other respiratory infections.

A small amount of fluid is present to lubricate this area to allow the lungs to "slide" along the chest wall during inhalation. If this area becomes inflamed, a sharp pain will be noticed during inhalation but not so much during exhalation. As the lung inflates it comes into contact with the irritated, less lubricated lining of the chest wall, causing a sharp pain. During exhalation, as the lung is deflating, contact and resultant friction is reduced and there is less or no noticeable pain.

Unless there are other underlying conditions, treatment is largely symptomatic. Breathing may be less painful while lying on the affected side. However, if breathing is already limited and the ability to take even a normal inhalation is compromised because of pain, seek medical attention before breathing becomes worse.

Pleural effusion is an excess of fluid between the layers of tissue that line the lungs and chest wall cavity. **Effusion** simply means an escape of fluid into a body cavity. This could be normal bodily fluids or infectious material. Normally only a small amount of fluid lines the pleural space to lubricate and reduce the friction as the lung expands along the chest wall. Excessive amounts of fluid will occupy the space and exert pressure inward. Since the ribs prevent the pressure from pressing outward, the only distortion will be inward, compressing the lung. Again, the ability to inhale will be limited because of this mechanical restriction.

Shortness of breath is likely to occur because of the inability to inhale deeply. Chest pain, coughing and a fever may also be noted, depending on the cause of the effusion. A smaller amount of fluid is able to be reabsorbed on its own. However, if fluid is excessive, a **thoracentesis** procedure may be performed by the doctor. A needle is inserted between the ribs into the pleural space to drain the fluid. The needle does not enter the lung. Depending on the analysis of the aspirated fluids, antibiotics or other therapy would be started as indicated.

Pulmonary nodules and other spots: Scar tissue normally forms as a result of healing. We are familiar with what happens with a cut on the skin that knits back together. A slight scar from the healing of the opposing edges often results. Lung tissue is no different and the healing process may have left some scar tissue that ultimately shows up on the x-ray. Micro scars are not uncommon in a normal chest x-ray and do not normally affect lung function. They are not necessarily indicators of chronic lung disease or even cancer. However, when the doctor mentions that the recent chest x-ray showed a "spot," the anxiety alarm bells ring. Let's look at a few of those terms consider their importance.

Pulmonary nodules are seen as a small round or oval-shaped shadows or spots on the x-ray. They are found in about half of all routine chest x-rays or CT scans and are more common with age. Nodules that are less than one inch in diameter are usually benign and are the result of tissue healing following an infection. Depending on medical history and accompanying symptoms, the doctor may recommend **watchful**

waiting. This simply means that chest x-rays will be repeated at specific intervals. If the nodule remains unchanged, for a year or two, no further therapy or monitoring is indicated.

Nodules that are larger than that are often referred to as a **lung mass** and may need to be investigated further. The larger nodules do not necessarily indicate malignancy. Depending on histories and clinical symptoms, a biopsy may be requested. Microscopic examination will more accurately determine if it is malignant or benign.

Granulomas can form anywhere in the body and often do so in response to an infection. **Macrophages** are white blood cells that engulf and digest cellular debris or foreign substances. If they are unable to eliminate the organism or foreign body, they may encompass it to wall it off from other tissue. Granulomas will be more noticeable later in life as calcium deposits accumulate. They usually are benign and unless there is a diagnosable cause, no treatment is required.

Neoplasm is an abnormal growth in or on the lung. The size is variable and often irregular in shape. Environmental exposures such as smoke, radon gas and asbestos often draw suspicion as to origin; however, a biopsy is usually needed for a more definitive diagnosis. The neoplasm may be benign, pre-cancerous or malignant. Although there are numerous causes for these abnormal growths, therapy will be customized to respond to that particular group of cells. An **oncologist** who specializes in the treatment of cancer will recommend the appropriate therapy. Surgery, chemotherapy, radiation or a combination may be suggested and tailor-made for the best therapeutic advantage.

Advances in the treatment of cancer have produced better results with fewer complications. Rather than a chemotherapy cocktail, drugs and doses are able to be used for specific cancers with individual calibrated doses to limit unpleasant side effects. Gene therapy is useful in some cancers. Specific enzymes are placed in cancer cells to make them more susceptible to particular chemotherapy agents. Advances in radiation technology have allowed for direct radiation of the tumor and reduced harmful exposure of non-involved tissue. Minimal invasive surgery is more often an option. Improvement in imaging techniques allows for laser-guided resection as well as the use of robotic instrumentation for smaller incisions. In some cases, immunotherapy has proven successful in utilizing the body's own immune system to destroy the tumor. A technique called **adoptive cell therapies** actually reengineers the white blood cells to fight specific cancers.

Although discovery of a malignant neoplasm is scary, the odds of survival are better now than they ever were.

These are just a few of the things that can complicate breathing.

Chronic lung disease doesn't necessarily mean that one will be constantly plagued with all that goes around. It does mean, however, that care must be taken. Pay attention to your surroundings, especially during cold and flu season, when exposure to viruses can escalate into more problems for those with preceding conditions. In this age of modern medicine where there is a cure for just about anything, prevention is still the best course of action. As my father used to remind me, rather than chasing the cows out of the cornfield, it's more effective to just keep the barn door closed.

Additional Reading

"Pneumonia," 13 July 2020, www.mayoclinic.org.
J. Christensen, February 2020, "Corona Virus Explained: What You Need to Know," www.cnn/2020/01/2020/health/what-is-covid-explained.
"Understanding Influenza Viruses," 10 July 2019, www.cdc.gov.
"Pulmonary Fibrosis," www.mayoclinic.org.

14

What About Other
Non-Infectious Problems?

In the previous chapter the emphasis was on those *tiny* germs that can cause *big* problems. Unintentional encounters with these germs have always been a fact of life. However, with chronic lung disease, a new level of caution and care is needed. But what about some of those other problems that we hear about from time to time? How are they related to chronic lung disease? Let's take a look at what one needs to know and diminish the chance that these conditions don't compound already troubled breathing.

Atelectasis is a condition in which some of the alveoli have collapsed and are unable to participate in proper gas exchange with the blood. This could be limited to patchy areas throughout the lungs or involve an entire lobe or more. Unlike an active infection, atelectasis is the result of decreased movement of air through the lungs. Excessive congestion, as a result of an upper respiratory infection, can temporarily block the smaller bronchial tubes. This will prevent aeration of alveoli beyond the mucus plug. Vigorous coughing usually remedies the blockage, restoring ventilation to the affected area.

Atelectasis is one of the most common complications following any type of surgery, especially abdominal or chest surgery. Early in the recovery the ability to be out of bed and move around is somewhat limited. Monitoring wires and drainage tubes aside, the need for pain management is the most obvious reason. Although rest and pain management are important, the lungs still operate on the basic principle of "use it or lose it." If breathing is shallow and air isn't being directed to the lower airways, the alveoli will eventually collapse.

Surfactant is a substance that lines the inside of the alveoli and reduces surface tension to prevent the lungs from collapsing. Moist surfaces, such as the alveoli, have an adhesive attraction. Surfactant disrupts this attraction to keep the alveoli open. During the normal breathing cycle, the alveoli are partially compressed on exhalation and re-expanded during inhalation. This action stimulates the release and recycling of surfactant. Although there are several physiologic stimuli responsible for maintaining surfactant's ability to work, intermittent deep inspiratory breaths are an important part. This is often referred to as a sigh or a yawn and normally occurs around a dozen times each hour. A sigh may be consciously noticed following a period of inactivity or when first waking. However, even when one is up and active, the need for periodically increasing the depth of breathing is necessary to keep surfactant viable. Fortunately, just the act of getting up from a chair and moving around a bit causes a change in inhaled volume and is a sufficient substitute for a sigh.

Hospitalized patients are encouraged to be out of bed as soon as is clinically appropriate. Coughing and deep breathing are constantly encouraged. Following abdominal surgery, one would think that coughing and movement would be the last thing that should be encouraged. Actually, it's one of the most important steps toward recovery. Mucus continues to be normally produced. The cilia which sweep it to the upper airways are slowed because of reduced activity. After a day or so, congestion will necessitate more vigorous coughing, unfortunately resulting in additional discomfort.

A device called an incentive spirometer is placed at the bedside for use. This device will not strengthen the lungs, as is often stated. It serves as a reminder to take the deep breaths and keep the surfactant viable. Just because the incentive spirometer was inadvertently moved beyond reach, deep breaths can still be taken. The spirometer also measures the depth of the inhalation. Without this visual input, the depth may actually be decreasing over several days without anyone even realizing it. The important point here is, following any surgery or prolonged illness, to

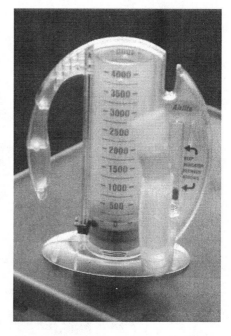

Incentive Spirometry (Johntex).

follow the instructions of the doctors, nurses and respiratory therapists. Prevention of atelectasis is much easier than the cure.

Obstructive sleep apnea (OSA) is one of the most underdiagnosed problems affecting the adult population today. More than 18 million Americans have been diagnosed and another estimated 10 million remain undiagnosed. Patients with OSA may stop breathing for over a minute at a time and do so 6 to 30+ times per hour. During these periods of **apnea** (*a* = prefix meaning "absence of"; *pnea* = "breathing") the muscles of the chest and diaphragm continue to flex in an attempt to move air. Unfortunately, the obstruction occurs in the back of the throat, blocking the movement of air into the lungs. COPD doesn't necessarily increase the chance of developing OSA but in some situations the problems can overlap. Essentially, when one's breathing is already compromised, one doesn't need any additional problems with it.

Normally, even while sleeping, there remains a slight muscle tone to the muscles in the neck. This tone keeps the tongue and other soft tissue from blocking the airway. However, during the deepest levels of sleep, **rapid eye movement (REM)** all of the skeletal muscles are temporarily paralyzed and this muscle tone is lost. As a result, if there is an excess of soft tissue in this area, obstruction many occur. During the obstruction, oxygen levels drop and levels of carbon dioxide increase. Once the brain detects these changes, arousal occurs and sleep becomes less deep and is often punctuated with a loud snore, snort or choking sound. Within a minute or so, REM sleep has resumed and the obstruction routine begins all over again.

Upon awakening in the morning, the patient may be unaware of these events that occurred during the night. However, their spouse will probably have a different story. In fact, most patients with significant OSA deny any sleep problems at all. "I can fall asleep anytime," they say. And unfortunately, that's true and it doesn't work out too well when one is driving. An estimated 30% of all traffic accidents are directly or indirectly the result of sleep deprivation.

Excessive daytime sleepiness may be an obvious symptom but so are morning headaches. Excessive accumulation of carbon dioxide causes blood vessels in the brain to dilate and the buildup of pressure results in an early morning headache.

Many undiagnosed OSA sufferers blame their sleepiness on frequent trips to the bathroom during the night. Although there may be various causes for this, OSA may also be a factor. As the diaphragm continues to flatten during inhalation, the downward pressure is also exerted on the bladder. This results in a squeezing of the bladder, signaling the brain that it's full and needs to be emptied. During REM sleep an "anti-diuretic" hormone is released which decreases the signals that the bladder is full. When REM sleep is interrupted, the anti-diuretic hormone may not be sufficient to discourage the sensation of a full bladder. There are also several other hormones that are only released during REM sleep that regulate the immune system. As a result, the lack of quality (REM) sleep will do more than cause daytime sleepiness; it's putting the patient at a higher risk for illness.

It's not too difficult to suspect that many (but certainly not all) patients who are significantly overweight may be at risk for OSA. Usually OSA has been experienced for about 10 years before it is diagnosed. Most people naturally assume that their pattern of sleep is normal for them. It's important to note, however, that neither snoring nor the absence of snoring are sufficient for diagnosing or dismissing the prospects of one's having OSA. Since the obstructed airway occurs in the back of the throat, nasal strips, though popular and advertised to stop snoring, will not prevent or treat OSA.

If OSA is suspected, talk with the doctor about being tested. The testing may require an overnight stay in a sleep lab; however, some labs may be able to allow one to self administer the test at home. If treatment is needed, there are several options available that are easily managed. CPAP is a device that delivers exactly what the name implies: continuous positive airway pressure. A small compressor generates air pressure that splints open the upper airways in the back of the throat. A BiPAP (bilevel positive airway pressure) device offers the same therapy but is calibrated for a slightly higher pressure upon inhalation and slightly less during exhalation. The difference is largely a matter of comfort. These devices offer therapy, not a cure. They are not difficult to use and there are various mask attachments and nasal pillows that fit into the nostril. The CPAP technology is also useful for some patients without OSA but are in the later stages of emphysema. The mild inspiratory pressure assumes partial work of breathing and, to a certain extent, provides a partial rest to those accessory muscles of respiration. It is not used as a ventilator, but merely as a temporary reprieve to the work of breathing.

Becoming adjusted is usually a matter of trial and error before one finds the most comfortable interface. The key here is don't give up. Correcting the effects of chronic sleep apnea is important, otherwise the doctor wouldn't have ordered it. If experiencing difficulty adjusting, call the home medical equipment supplier and ask to try a different mask. It's their job to make this system work for you. But most importantly remember that a good night's sleep is fundamental to managing one's health. Let's look at a few more examples of non-infectious diseases and recommended actions.

Congestive heart failure (CHF) is a failure of the heart muscle to adequately pump blood. It doesn't mean that the heart isn't working anymore, just that it's now pumping blood through the body at a much lower volume. Oxygen and other vital nutrients therefore may not be delivered fast enough to meet the body's demands. The most common causes of CHF are cardiovascular disease such as a heart attack, hypertension, hypothyroid, anemia and diabetes. Although there are many reasons why this may occur, patients with chronic low oxygen levels are also at a greater risk for developing CHF.

Let's use the example of obstructive sleep apnea, discussed a moment ago. If the lungs are falling down on the job, the heart has to pick up the slack and pump harder. Many patients have a long-standing problem of snoring, sputtering and gasping during sleep. They may not arouse or are even be aware of what's happening but while sleeping, their oxygen levels vary from high to low as if the track of a roller coaster. While the body is sleeping and trying to rest, the poor heart is working overtime. The heart is a muscle and any muscle worked harder tends to get bigger. And at first this is an advantage, since a bigger heart muscle pumps more blood. Oxygen gets where it's needed and everybody's happy. Unfortunately, over the years, as this is going on night after night, the heart finally reaches a size that is just too large and overstretched. Its size now limits its ability to contract with enough force to expel sufficient blood with each stroke. A volume of blood remains in the left ventricle following each contraction. This causes a dilation of the left ventricle. It's like a piece of elastic stretched a little, a big snap. Stretched a little farther, a bigger snap. Eventually the elastic is stretched too far and doesn't return to its original shape. Overstretching of the heart is known as **cardiomegaly**, or enlargement of the heart. Now none of the body's parts are getting the blood and oxygen they need, and shortness of breath becomes an early symptom.

Swelling (**edema**), especially of the feet and legs, is also noticed. As less blood is being pumped, the kidneys misinterpret this as low blood volume. The high priority of the kidneys is to manage fluid levels and maintain adequate blood pressure. Their response will be to immediately start retaining fluids. Although the kidneys are performing as they should, unfortunately they're acting on the wrong information. There's plenty of fluid in the vascular system and that retained fluid has to go somewhere. Since the blood vessels can only hold so much, the retained fluid is pressed into the surrounding tissue and first noticed in the lower extremities. While one is standing or sitting with the legs down, gravity is competing with the failing heart in pumping the blood back up to the heart for recirculation. Swelling of the lower extremities with edema is easily noticed. If not soon corrected, fluid retention will progressively move upward. As the tissue in the abdominal area becomes saturated, breathing will be noticeably difficult. If left unchecked, the excess fluid will push into the alveoli, resulting in **pulmonary edema**, a serious, life-threatening event.

Obviously, sitting with the feet elevated helps relieve the edema but that's only a temporary solution. Managing fluid intake and urine output on a daily basis is critical. Using a typical bathroom scale, monitor your weight every morning. The goal isn't to lose body fat, it's to make sure body weight from fluid stays within acceptable limits. Normally, an adult's weight fluctuates by several pounds each day, but noticing an upward trend, several days in a row, indicates that fluid is being retained. Have an action plan worked out with the doctor and already in place so the necessary changes can be made before the accumulated fluid becomes a real emergency. Don't wait till your feet look like basketballs and breathing is difficult to start worrying about it. Daily weight monitoring is key.

Gastroesophageal reflux disease syndrome (GERDS) isn't exactly a lung disease but it can result in significant respiratory problems. Remember the normal upper airway anatomy and how the esophagus (swallowing tube) and trachea (breathing tube) have a common area in the throat? And remember those nights when going to bed late after eating one too many slices of pepperoni pizza and later were jolted awake with "heartburn"? Fortunately, this didn't have anything to do with the heart, it was more likely excessive stomach acid creeping back up the esophagus causing a burning pain. The esophagus is a durable tube and able to handle spicy foods and liquids going down it. Stomach acids coming back up the wrong way, however, is another story. Strong stomach acid is very irritating and the result is the discomfort described as heartburn because it's in the middle of the chest. It is possible for a small amount of that acid to actually reach the opening of the esophagus and be aspirated into the trachea. Remember how delicate the tissue of the trachea is, and the resultant violent coughing if even a little bit of anything goes "down the wrong pipe"? It's not too hard to imagine how much damage some of this stomach acid will do to the trachea. Occasionally patients who never smoked and have no history of exposure to environmental hazards are diagnosed with chronic bronchitis as a result of chronic GERDS. For many asthmatics, nighttime asthma attacks can be triggered by GERDS.

Medication is often prescribed to lessen the amount of acid produced. However, many patients have reduced the incidence of GERDS by raising the head of their beds by about 4 inches. The stomach sphincter is located where the esophagus meets the stomach. Acid is a liquid, and while one is lying flat, is more likely to seek the level of the sphincter and enter the esophagus. Raising the head of the bed about four inches (not just the pillows) may increase the angle necessary to reduce the incidence of reflux. A distended abdomen will be compressed when lying on one's side. This may be enough to push the stomach acid up to the sphincter. Common sense also applies here; eating or drinking large amounts of spicy foods before going to bed should be avoided.

Pulmonary artery hypertension (PAH) is a type of high blood pressure that affects the arteries of the lungs and the right ventricle of the heart. PAH is not the same as regular high blood pressure. If the tiny arteries in the lungs become narrowed, blocked or destroyed, blood flow through the lungs is slowed. As the right ventricle of the heart continues to push blood into these affected arteries, the increased resistance raises the pressure in the lung's arteries. As a result, constant back pressure on the right ventricle causes it to stretch or dilate. There are numerous causes for PAH, including congestive heart failure, blood clots in the lungs, autoimmune diseases as well as others. Included in this list are chronic lung disease, sleep apnea and pulmonary fibrosis. Since lower levels of oxygen are the common factor, let's expand a little on why this may happen.

Prior to birth, our lungs aren't being used and lower amounts of oxygen are provided by the placenta. Although the oxygen concentration is low, it is sufficient. Since the lungs aren't being used, blood flow was largely shunted around them. The lower oxygen content is responsible for limiting the blood circulation to the lungs. At birth, when the umbilical cord is clamped and the first several breaths are taken, the oxygen levels sharply increase. The clamping of the cord and increased oxygen open up the blood vessels in the lungs. With that being said, when blood oxygen levels again are low, for whatever reason, the physiology of the lungs and circulatory system tend to revert back to this earlier pathway. It would only seem logical that lower oxygen levels would expand the blood flow to the lungs, but that isn't the case. When aeration to various lung compartments is unavailable or reduced, blood flow will be **shunted** to other portions of the lung where gas exchange is able to occur. The body is trying to remedy what is called a **ventilation/perfusion mismatch** (air/blood mismatch).

Diagnostic tests such as echocardiograms and CT scans can check for indications of increased pressures in the pulmonary arteries. An ECG can show if the right side of the heart is under strain. A cardiac stress test can measure oxygen levels and heart and lung function during exercise. These may ultimately determine the need for a right heart catheterization for more definitive information.

With patients with a history of chronic lung disease, especially in later stages, most doctors will focus on correcting the low oxygen levels as opposed to more definitive diagnostic testing. The important point here is that if oxygen therapy is recommended, use it. If therapy for sleep apnea, such as CPAP or BiPAP, is recommended, use it. Dietary recommendations to manage salt and fluid intake need to be followed.

Pulmonary fibrosis is scarring of the lungs in the lower airways and most significantly at the alveolar level. It is a restrictive disease (rather than obstructive like COPD) and limits the ability to expand the lungs adequately during inhalation. The sensation of a restrictive lung disease would be similar to a belt being placed around the chest, restricting expansion. The stiffness caused by the scar tissue limits the ability to inhale much more than a normal size breath. As a result, shortness of breath is noticeable even with mild exertion. Very often the first symptom of pulmonary fibrosis is a dry hacking cough whenever a deeper breath is attempted. Normally **stretch receptors** in the lung tissue limit an active inhalation. When the stretch limits are reached an exhalation is signaled. In other words, it's not possible to simply keep inhaling until the lungs pop like a balloon. When excessive scar tissue is present, the stretch receptors reach their end point at a much lower volume, resulting in a cough.

The second problem is the ability to move gases between the lungs and blood. Normally the alveoli are very thin air sacs, but when scar tissue forms, the alveoli become thickened and stiff. Since oxygen and carbon dioxide pass (**diffuse**) through this membrane, the thicker it is, the slower the movement across the alveoli. Think of how a glass of water poured into a small paper sack will dribble out rather quickly. However, if poured into five or six paper sacks stacked inside one another, water would still dribble out but it would take much longer to do so. And that's the major problem with pulmonary fibrosis, the slow exchange of gas between the alveoli and the blood circulation.

Scar tissue forms as the result of healing following an injury or infection. Although everyone does have some scar tissue in their lungs, pulmonary fibrosis interferes with breathing when it is more generalized through a large area of the lungs. Chest x-rays may detect some fibrous areas but a biopsy would be needed to more accurately determine the diagnosis. During early stages, management is largely supportive to maintain oxygen levels as necessary. In later stages, lung transplants are often recommended as scar tissue does not go away.

About 40% of all pulmonary fibrosis diagnosis are classified as

idiopathic, which is the medical term for "cause is undetermined." There are, however, several likely causes. A genetic link is suspected in that certain people have a predisposition for extensive scar formation. A history of prolonged untreated GERDS, frequent lung infections and occupational exposures to silica and coal dust as well as asbestosis fibers are thought to be contributing factors. However, many with a history of one or other of the above factors do not develop fibrosis. Radiation therapy has been suspected but other patients with similar exposures don't develop fibrosis. Some medications have also been linked to increasing the chance of developing significant pulmonary fibrosis. That's why it is important to read those warning labels on any new medicine and talk with the doctor and pharmacist about any concerns. If pulmonary fibrosis is noted in the warning section, discuss the risks vs. benefits with the doctor. A pulmonary function that includes **diffusion capacity (DLCO)** should be done prior to or soon after starting any new medicines in which a concern about pulmonary fibrosis is listed. The DLCO (**diffusion lung carbon monoxide**) is a measure of the movement of gas across the alveoli and provides a baseline study for comparison. This screening should be reexamined and monitored every six months as long as that particular medicine is continued.

Spontaneous pneumothorax may occur as a result of a ruptured alveoli that allows air from the alveoli to leak into the pleural space between the lung and chest wall. As pressure builds, the affected lung is squeezed inward, compressing the remaining air spaces. Breathing becomes progressively (and rapidly) more difficult. The ruptured alveoli may act as a one-way valve, allowing air into the pleural space but not back into the alveoli. As pressure continues to build between the chest wall and lung, the trapped air pushes the affected lung against the heart, limiting its ability to function properly. This is called a **tension pneumothorax** and is a true medical emergency.

Overstretched alveoli that have formed large **blebs** may rupture following an episode of forceful coughing. Although the possibility of a pneumothorax are increased with severe emphysema, the occurrence is infrequent. Symptoms include sudden onset of chest pain on the affected side and shortness of breath. Medical attention is needed as soon as possible.

Obviously, chest trauma such as a punctured chest wall from a penetrating chest wound, or a broken rib pushed inward and puncturing the lung will necessitate a trip to the emergency room. If a significant volume of the lung is being compressed a chest tube may be inserted into the pleural space to remove the excessive air from the pleural space. The tube would be placed in the pleural space and would not enter the lung.

This would require hospitalization and could take several days for suffi-cient air to be evacuated. The tear in the alveoli will normally heal shut, and after a few days and the chest tube will then be removed.

Smaller volumes of trapped air that are causing distress may be removed with a needle aspiration without the need of a chest tube. Although this may be done as a bedside procedure, close supervision for a day or so is often recommended to ensure that air doesn't reen-ter the pleural space. A smaller pneumothorax that doesn't appear to be increasing in size and not significantly limiting breathing may simply be closely monitored for a few days while allowing the air to reabsorb.

Bronchiectasis, although an obstructive lung disease, is not clas-sified as COPD and is not related to bronchitis. The term uses the com-bining form **bronchi-** (pertaining to the descending, progressively smaller, bronchial tubes) and the noun **ectasis**, meaning expansion. This is a permanent enlargement of parts of the smaller airways. Respira-tory infections are more common with this condition because the pool-ing of mucus provides germs with an ideal warm, moist environment in which to grow. The cilia are overwhelmed due to the accumulated local volume. Frequent productive coughing and respiratory infections are prominent. Bronchiectasis most often occurs as a result of frequent and prolonged respiratory infections resulting in chronic inflammation of the airways. This is termed **acquired bronchiectasis**. The chronic inflammation weakens the structure of the bronchial wall, resulting in dilation. **Congenital bronchiectasis** may be present at birth and is more often the result of other inherited medical problems such as **cys-tic fibrosis**. Conditions that limit the cilias' ability to clear the airways properly or dramatically affect the production of mucus are contrib-uting factors. Smoking is generally not a causative issue, since limited breathing and coughing are often progressive from childhood. Bronchi-ectasis patients simply can't afford any more complications with breath-ing, so smoking is not usually attempted. Surgical resection was once recommended but today's improved antibiotics and physiotherapy tech-niques to promote bronchial drainage are usually adequate.

While increasing awareness about breathing and how the body functions, one will likely encounter references to many of these condi-tions. A better understanding of what's going on will hopefully decrease one's anxiety and improve communication with one's health care team. A history of chronic lung disease doesn't necessarily mean that one will develop any of these conditions. It does mean, however, that care must be taken. The health care team is there to help. Make sure their instruc-tions and advice are understood and followed. And by all means, avoid first- or even secondhand smoke. I sincerely hope that smoking isn't a problem for you, but if it is, this next chapter may be the most important one. Let's turn the page and start finding a solution—for yourself or a loved one.

Additional Reading

Timothy J. Legg, MD, CRNP, 19 June 2020, "Everything to Know about the 5 Stages of Sleep," www.healthline.com.
Jennifer Warner, 25 July 2008, "Link Found Between Asthma and GERDs," www.webMD.com.
"Obstructive Sleep Apnea," www.mayoclinic.org.
"Chest X-Rays," www.mayoclinic.org.
"Heart Failure," www.mayoclinic.org.

15

Still Smoking
After All These Years?

I sincerely hope this is one chapter that can be skipped. Unfortunately, I've met a lot of folks devastated by COPD who just can't seem to kick the habit. Rationalizations such as "One every now and then won't hurt me," and of course, "The damage is already done, so what's the use?" I interviewed one man who was tethered to his oxygen tank but still needed his morning cigarette with his cup of coffee. "I have a 50-foot oxygen hose so, to be safe, I leave the oxygen tank on the other side of the room while I smoke." I pointed out to him that the oxygen was still coming out the cannula in his nose. "Oh," he said, suddenly realizing the implication of my comment, "maybe that's why they burn up so fast!"

Even if you have been successful at quitting, you may know a few others, perhaps family or friends, who haven't yet felt the need to quit or tried and failed. Helping them find a way to quit before they get to the point where you may now find yourself could be a blessing in disguise.

A history of smoking becomes more significant once it approaches what's called the **20 pack-year** mark. That's an average of 1 pack per day (PPD) for 20 years. Of course, multiples of this, i.e., 2 PPD for 10 years, also apply, so do the math. Fortunately, only about 30% of smokers will eventually have significant breathing problems. However, anyone approaching this benchmark will more than likely be noticing some breathing limitations. Obviously, genetics, aging and occupational exposures also play a significant role in the development and severity of chronic lung disease.

It was once widely thought that just smoking less would be helpful in reducing lung damage due to cigarette use, but research has proven otherwise. **Carbon monoxide (CO)** is the result of incomplete combustion, which is why there's smoke. CO is inhaled with each drag and binds tightly to the oxygen-carrying red blood cells, displacing oxygen.

Carbon monoxide remains bound to the hemoglobin for several hours after just one cigarette. As a result, for the next several hours, the ability to carry oxygen is reduced up to 7%. That may be fine if one's oxygen saturation is near 100% to begin with. Tolerating a little shortness of breath may not be a big deal, but why risk it? However, what if one's oxygen saturations are only in the low 90s to begin with? Remember how the respiratory therapist grows concerned when one's oxygen saturations are reading in the low to mid–80s? Just smoke one cigarette and subtract 7% from 85% and see what happens. And no matter how many inhalers puffs are taken, they aren't going to bring one's oxygen levels back to where they were before that cigarette. It takes several hours.

Unfortunately, the delicate bronchial tubes also take a big hit in the form of irritation. Increased mucus and inflammation, which further narrow the diameter in which air must flow, also limit breathing. An older doctor once explained it to me this way: "If you had a small cut on your arm, and you cleaned it and left it alone, it would scab over in a day or so and heal up. But, if every day, you spent five minutes rubbing it with your hand and irritating that cut, would it ever heal up?" Of course not. The tenderness of the bronchial tubes is no different. They will respond to that irritation, which will consequently obstruct breathing. So, no, cutting down doesn't work out in the long run. *But it's a start.*

Those of us who quit smoking 30-plus years ago, when **cold turkey** was the only option, know that it's not an easy road. Mark Twain put it well when he said, "Quitting smoking was the easiest thing I have ever done; I've quit thousands of times." And he was right. Nicotine is one of the most addictive substances known to man. None of us were born smokers; it is a learned behavior and everyone begins smoking for their own reasons. If friends smoked, the pressure to share a common bond was difficult to rebuff. Unfortunately, as the years rolled on, smoking became a larger part of one's life, until eventually smoking became a necessity, not an option.

Fortunately, today those making an attempt to quit have a lot more help available than ever before. Although the advertisements make it sound easy, make no mistake, quitting isn't as easy as just slapping on a patch or popping a pill. Most people make at least half a dozen attempts before successfully quitting. If, however, your attempts to kick the habit have been unsuccessful, let's explore, a little deeper, the science of quitting.

There are two aspects to quitting smoking, and both have to be dealt with in order for one to succeed: **addiction to nicotine** and the **associated behavioral aspects**. Let's first look at nicotine and what it does. Remember the earlier discussion of medications and the receptors that they stimulate? The chemicals that carry the message to a particular receptor are called **neurotransmitters**. Nicotine rapidly stimulates the release of the neurotransmitter **epinephrine** (more commonly known as **adrenaline**). This rapidly constricts the blood vessels and increases the heart rate, both of which increase blood pressure. The increased blood pressure to the brain improves alertness. As a result, if one is feeling sad, tired or bored, nicotine will perk one right up. If, however, when one is feeling overly stimulated—just wound too tight—smoking can have a calming, relaxing effect. This paradoxical effect is most likely due to the act of smoking itself and not nicotine, since one normally has to "slow down" to smoke. Nicotine and the act of smoking, therefore, are kind of like a good friend, always meeting those needs, no matter what they are.

The addictive aspects of nicotine take a slightly different pathway. Nicotine increases the release of **dopamine**, another neurotransmitter, which affects the reward pathways, also known as the pleasure receptors of the brain. Another neurotransmitter, **glutamate**, is released, which enhances connection with the memory and learning centers of the brain, reinforcing a memory loop. And of course, if pleasurable responses are learned, addiction becomes much more likely. Even though everyone knows that smoking is harmful, this learned memory loop helps one come up with any number of excuses why "I'll quit one of these days, just not today."

In addition to nicotine, cigarette smoke contains hundreds of other compounds unfavorable to good health. Most notable is **tar**, which is the product of burning tobacco. This is the substance that temporarily paralyzes the respiratory cilia which assist with secretion removal. Tar is the substance most closely associated with lung damage, including cancer. Filtered cigarettes were introduced to help remove some of the inhaled tar from burning tobacco. Unfortunately, only a small portion is trapped, the rest is inhaled into the lungs and accumulates. Rather than appearing a healthy *pinkish*, the lungs of a chronic smoker will appear *grayish*. Tobacco products are rated relative to the amount of tar produced: *low-tar, mild, light* and *ultra-light*. Unfortunately, there is no safe cigarette. Smokers of ultra-light cigarettes will tend to inhale more deeply and more often than smokers of non-filtered cigarettes.

Okay, cold turkey has been tried again and again with little to no success. Now it's time to step it up a bit. The first thing is to discover when and why smoking is needed. Below is a simple little chart that can be of use in helping one to understand their own need to smoke. Use this as a survey and make one page for each day. A week's worth of information is usually enough, since there may be some days (such as the weekend) where the daily routine may be significantly different. In the first column of the chart (*Time*), record the time whenever you light up. It doesn't matter if just one drag was taken or it was smoked to the filter, just write down the time. Next, check the box in the next three columns (*Needed*) that best describes how badly the cigarette was needed at that particular moment. In the last three columns (*Mood*), check the box that best indicates your mood when lighting up: in a good mood, happy and upbeat; or bored and tired, or in a gloomy downbeat mood.

After a week, sit down and analyze the results. First of all, look for patterns. There will be patterns in the times when you were smoking and not smoking. Also, patterns when several cigarettes were smoked in a short span and other parts of the day when smoking didn't occur at all. Some of these patterns may simply be the result of opportunities such as a consistent break at work or other times when one is unable to smoke because of time or place. It's quite likely that most days will show a similar pattern. Next, the *Need* columns will help one identify the instances of smoking that one might have eliminated without really missing them. The three *Mood* columns help to identify the reasons for smoking. Everyone has their individual reasons for smoking, and quitting will also be an individual process. Given that smoking can speed things up or calm them down, it's important to know the reason (desire) for smoking. If nicotine is being used as a reward, such as for finishing a task, find another reward system. If it's used because you are bored, find something else to occupy your attention. If tired, take a nap, but if that's not practical, go for a walk or something else to get the blood pressure up instead of using nicotine to do it. If depressed, sad or angry, talk with the doctor about other options. There are much safer and less expensive options available.

If, for the last several months smoking occurred less than ten times each day and the majority of *Need* selections in your week's results were in the first two columns, you're ready to begin the process of quitting. If,

	TIME	Need:	NEED:	**NEED:**	Mood :)	MOOD < * * >	**MOOD :(**
	of lighting up	would like one	Yes - soon	**RIGHT NOW**	Happy & up-beat	Bored & Tired	Depressed, or angry
1							
2							
3							
4							
5							
etc							

Smoking needs scale.

however, the majority of *Need* selections were in the "Right Now" column and *Mood* selection were in the "Angry or Depressed" column, talk with the doctor. One of the oral medications such as Wellbutrin (Zyban) or Chantix that are currently on the market may be helpful. Essentially, these medications help relieve some of the anxiety associated with nicotine withdrawal. Although they won't make one quit, they might help until one can better manage the need to smoke. Be honest when discussing this with the doctor. Depending on one's medical history or other medicines that might be needed, these products may not be safe. However, in individual cases, they can be very helpful. Use of these supplements may take several weeks to reduce the desire to smoke, so be patient. After several weeks, repeat the survey and hopefully there will be some changes noted from the previous smoking habit.

If one's daily consumption averages well over one pack per day, it might be useful to use **nicotine replacement therapy (NRT)**. There are several varieties available. Nicotine patches of 21 mg, 14 mg and 7 mg are available without prescription. If selecting a nicotine patch, chose a dose that's close to one's average daily need for nicotine. One pack of cigarettes is equivalent to about 20 mg of nicotine. I've said "about" because how deeply one inhales, the choice of cigarettes and how much of the cigarette is smoked all contribute to the dose of nicotine. It's not an exact science. However, if you are smoking well over a pack per day don't select one of the lower-dose patches. It won't meet your individual needs. Regardless of the patch selected, it is extremely important that one ***never, ever smoke while wearing a patch.*** Remember what nicotine does—increasing the heart rate and constricting the blood vessels; both of which raise blood pressure. The combined dose of nicotine could result in nicotine toxicity, which can have serious, and possibly fatal effects. Don't risk it. Additionally, the patch often causes skin irritation so follow directions and, when replacing the patch, move it to a different location each day. Disruption of sleep is also a common complication, since nicotine is not normally consumed while sleeping. It's recommended to remove the patch during normal sleep. After a few weeks, begin to reduce the dosage of nicotine.

Nicotine patches release their dose of nicotine at a set rate while worn. Looking back at the completed charts, one will notice that smoking is cyclic in nature. In other words, there are times when the dose of the nicotine patch will be sufficient, but other times when one will be under-dosed. This steady nicotine dosing rather than cyclic patterned smoking is usually the reason why many simply give up, saying, "I've tried but nothing worked." However, keep working at it. NRT is also available in chewing gum and lozenges in 1 mg or 2 mg dosages and are also over the counter. However, nicotine inhalers and nasal sprays require a prescription by a doctor. These mini-doses of nicotine may be helpful for those times when a "quick hit" is needed. In the past, perhaps you've tried and failed at using these nicotine replacement therapies. But most of the time failing is the result of not using them correctly or to the best advantage. We'll discuss the use of these supplements a little later. Remember, trying and failing isn't the same as giving up. When finding after a few weeks of NRT that consumption has been reduced to no more than one pack per day, it will become evident that you now have some control over nicotine rather than the other way around. There will always be those ups and downs, and just cutting down isn't the end goal, but it's a start.

During the last few years, **electronic cigarettes (e-cigarettes)** have become popular. Nicotine drops are added to a water cartridge which is heated up and releases a nicotine-laced vapor when inhaled. As with smoking a cigarette, the actual dosage is variable but an equivalent dose of about one to two cigarettes is delivered with each nicotine load. Be very careful not to overdo it as nicotine toxicity is still possible. The good news is that carbon monoxide and tar are not produced. As a result, there won't be any competition with the oxygen-carrying hemoglobin or buildup of tar in the lungs. The bad news, though, is the nicotine is addicting and causes harm by increasing the work the heart has to do. Additionally, flavor enhancers, often in the form of oils, may be added to the cartridge. These oils are heated, vaporized and inhaled into the lungs, where they cool and remain. As a result, some have been shown to cause additional health problems, which may be permanent and life-threatening.

There is a misconception that these devices can help one quit smoking. Unfortunately, the evidence points otherwise and many young adults are using e-cigarettes instead of tobacco and becoming addicted to nicotine. Switching from cigarettes to cigars or a pipe as a method of quitting was once thought to be a stepping-stone. Due to the methods of drying tobacco, cigarette smoke is more acidic and needs to be absorbed into the blood from the lungs. Tobacco used for pipe and cigar smoking is dried differently and is more alkaline and able to be absorbed in the mouth. Cigarette smokers switching to pipe or cigar tobacco will still have a tendency to inhale the smoke. As a result, switching methods of smoking is just a substitute and won't help reduce the need for nicotine. Carbon monoxide is still a by-product which interferes with the hemoglobin's ability to carry oxygen. As with cigarettes, nicotine is still absorbed with these products.

By now the survey has been completed (or perhaps repeated) and one now has a better idea of when and why smoking is needed. Now, it's time to get serious about quitting. All those boxes in the *Need* column that were marked "would like one"? Plan to eliminate them. After a week or so they are likely not to be missed anymore because that "friend" is still around when needed. After a week or two of eliminating those easy ones, consumption should be about half what it had been. Time to work on those in the second *Need* column: "Yes—soon." These will take a little more work.

Those nicotine receptors will be acting up a little more, wanting attention. However, if one doesn't surrender to the urge to smoke, those "nervous" nicotine receptors will actually back off in 7 to 10 minutes. Our nervous system is incapable of sustaining an increasing demand for very long and that's the average "attention span" (for lack of a more scientific term) for the nicotine receptors. Just fool them. When first inhaling a drag, there's an instant buzz, right? In all actuality, blood flow to the brain isn't instantaneous. The mechanism that causes this instant buzz is something that can be used to take the "edge" off. Part of that immediate response comes from a patch of nerves in the back of the throat. When stimulated by the irritating smoke, a biofeedback mechanism sends an instant message to the nicotine receptors in the brain and tells them: "Back off, boys, it's on the way." That patch of nerves in the back of the throat has learned, over the years of smoking, that the irritation of smoke means that nicotine is on the way down, and the initial response to nicotine begins. Try this; put a drinking straw between your lips and teeth and sharply inhale air through the straw a few times. The concentrated air stream will be sensed as "irritation" and send the message to the nicotine receptors. After a few minutes, when nicotine doesn't get to the brain, take a few more "air" hits. The straw also gives the hands something to do. The same effect can be produced by plugging one of the nostrils and inhaling sharply. Others have found that drinking water out of a bottle (not a glass) or peeling an orange and eating the slices one at a time have a similar effect. The citric acid of the orange and the movement of water against these nerve bundles are responsible. E-cigarettes without nicotine still release a vapor when inhaled that actually causes a similar response. Hopefully this will help you get through that 7- to 10-minute window.

For most, a common time of day to light up is following a meal. After we eat, food needs to be digested and enter the bloodstream. In order to expedite the process, the blood flow to the extremities (legs, arms and brain) is reduced and shifted to the gut to speed digestion. That's why we don't go swimming after eating; the legs cramp because of reduced blood flow, not the food. After eating, the blood flow to the brain also decreases, because the head is also an extension from the core. This causes the nicotine receptors in the brain to start getting nervous, "Hey, what about us?" Lighting up and taking that first drag speeds up the heart and the brain gets the blood flow it wants and everybody's happy. Therefore, change that behavior a little and instead of plopping down in an easy chair with a cup of coffee and lighting up, go for a walk. Do something to get the heart rate up a bit to keep the nicotine receptors happy with the blood flow. The same physiology holds true when one is first waking up or shortly before going to bed. It's "sluggish" blood flow to the brain, not the need for nicotine, that's driving the desire to light up.

Perhaps, though, that's not enough and "soon" keeps being pushed out until one gets to the "Right Now" column. That's where a little additional NRT might come in handy. **Nicotine gum, lozenges, inhalers or nasal sprays** may be helpful here. Taking a piece of nicotine gum and taking a few chomps to release a low dose of nicotine may be enough to get one over a rough spot without lighting up. With the nicotine gum, there is a method to using it: When chewing it, one will feel the "tingle" when nicotine is released. At that time, park the gum between the teeth and gum until another hit is needed. If one continuously chews the nicotine gum, too much nicotine will be released and nausea is likely. It would be like lighting up a cigarette and continuously taking drags until it's gone. Take it easy.

However, kicking the nicotine habit is only half the battle. Modifying those associated learned behavioral habits is the other. In fact, for many, that's the biggest part of the challenge. In view of the fact that nicotine stimulates the pleasurable receptors in the brain, any activities associated with smoking also get tied into this memory loop. If you are simply taking nicotine out of the common activity that has always been associated with smoking, it's going to be tough not to light up. Therefore, breaking this pattern of behavior will be necessary. Actually, men and women often smoke for different reasons: men to increase alertness and aggressiveness, women for social interaction. The next time you encounter a group of people on a smoke break, it's likely you'll see women in small groups of friends while the men are often off standing by themselves—they just need the nicotine. Therefore, while NRT may be more useful for men, behavioral modification may be more important for women. Make no mistake, though, attention to nicotine addiction and behavioral modification are important for both men and women.

How do we go about undoing all those things that we have associated with smoking over the years? It's not easy because it may not be possible to change all of those circumstances. If, however, one takes a closer look, a solution is likely to be found. Just a few tips that may be helpful:

- If your cigarettes are normally purchased by the carton, start buying them one pack at a time. The more trips one has to make to the store to stand in line, the more inconvenient it will be. And isn't that one of the things one needs to learn—that smoking is more of a hassle than it's worth?
- Don't buy your regular brand; buy a different kind. If normally a menthol smoker, buy non-menthol, or the other way around. Not that one is healthier than the other, but while continuing to smoke your favorite brand it will be harder to quit.
- Get rid of those objects normally associated with smoking such as ashtrays. Don't keep cigarettes within easy reach. If you have to walk out to the car, in the dark, when it's raining, just to get a cigarette, you might discover that it's just not worth it.
- Keep the lighter in a different (inconvenient) place than the cigarettes. Make a chore out of lighting up.
- Some over-the-counter throat lozenges and any hard candy with anise actually make cigarettes taste awful.
- Make a list of the reasons why quitting is important. Perhaps you have a picture of a loved one who is wanting you to quit. Keep it in a place where your cigarettes are normally kept. Now, when reaching for a smoke, that reminder of the need for quitting will be there.
- Let friends and family know that you're trying to quit. Social plans may need to be altered a bit because it will be hard to socialize with those you would normally smoke with. They'll understand and perhaps they'll join in the quest to quit.
- Support groups are available in most communities, and many people take comfort in knowing that others are fighting the same battle. If you need help finding a group, call the American Lung Association (1-800-LUNGUSA) to find a Better Breathers program available in your community.

Below are a few examples of what's worked for some of the patients I've known who were able to cut down but just had a hard time quitting those last few cigarettes each day:

- On her drive to and from work each day, Betty would light up as she left the driveway. Ten minutes later, when she entered the expressway, she lit up her second one. She couldn't smoke at work and the kids gave her too much grief to smoke at home, but the drive to and from work each day, over the same route, resulted in the same smoking pattern. "It was just automatic," she said. She started taking a slightly different route to work—breaking the pattern.

- Jim had worked as a consultant for years and much of his day involved talking on the phone. Every time he picked up the phone with his left hand, the right hand was ready with a cigarette. He started picking up the phone with his right hand—breaking the pattern.

- Eleanor and her husband had almost quit smoking but following their evening meal they would retire to the living room and watch the same nightly news. A couple of cigarettes became a normal part of that experience. Going for a short walk after supper instead of retiring to the living room was helpful, but the summer evenings were either too hot to be outdoors or late-afternoon thunderstorms would keep them in. On those occasions, they stayed home and watched the news but on a different channel—breaking the pattern.

- Robert was a tightwad. Not that he didn't have money; he did, he just didn't like to waste it. He had been a 2 PPD smoker for about 25 years and was able to get down to one cigarette in the morning and one at night, but couldn't get past that. He agreed that the best cigarette drag was the first from the first cigarette out of a brand-new pack. The agreement we made was that each morning and evening he could walk, *not* drive, to the 7-Eleven several blocks away and buy his favorite brand, open it, take one drag, then put it out and throw away the pack. He did that for about a week before finally deciding to quit for good—he couldn't waste that kind of money. Incidentally we later did come calculations and at an average of $5 per pack × 2 per day for 25 years, he had spent well over $91,000 on cigarettes.

Even though the progress of quitting seems to be on track, the battle isn't over yet. Those nicotine receptors may have been knocked down a peg or two but they don't just roll over like that. In fact the urge to resume smoking "just one" should be expected. Perhaps a feeling of "I've got this under control now; one will be OK." I've spoken with many who had quit for as long as five or six years, had a stressful moment, and started up again, just like they had never quit. It's an extremely hard habit to kick! But stick to it. It's an ongoing battle.

Remember that everyone began smoking for their own reasons, so finding a way to live without the need for nicotine is an individual process. Quitting techniques that worked for one may not work for someone else. When learning to smoke, it wasn't easy at first. Coughing and spitting were part of the process. After a while, those side effects became part of the daily routine and weren't so noticeable anymore. Now learning not to smoke will present a new set of challenges, and it won't be easy at first; it takes a lot of determination and effort but it can be done. If trying to quit, stick with it. If it's a loved one who's trying to quit, give them support—don't nag.

I sincerely hope this chapter has offered some insight into the science of smoking and nicotine addiction. Fortunately, smoking today is less acceptable now than it was in the past. Just watch an older movie from the 1950s or so: everyone was smoking. That's not the way it is now but smoking continues to be a health concern for millions. Teens experimenting with electronic cigarettes still submit themselves to the serious hazards of nicotine. So, the battle continues. If not for yourself, perhaps this chapter could help a loved one find their way to smoking cessation.

The next chapter may offer a template of sorts for those who need to begin this journey. But in all actuality, if a change or modification in behavior is identified, for any of the topics that have been discussed, perhaps the provided goals worksheet will help identify a path forward.

Additional Reading

Carly Vandergriendt, 3 January 2020, "Is Vaping Bad for You? and 12 Other FAQs," www.healthline.com.
"Quit Smoking: 10 tips," 2 March 2018, www.hopkinsmedicine.org.
"Smoking and Respiratory Diseases," www.hopkinsmedicine.org.

16

How Can I Put
This All Together
and Make It Work?

It's scary when the diagnosis of chronic lung disease is first learned. The doctor briefly explains that there is no cure but then says, "Here are a few things that might help." And it's particularly scary when shortness of breath reoccurs time and again and things seem to be spiraling out of control. Looking back at workplace exposures and lifestyle choices ("If only I would have...") offers only frustration. However, the path to regaining some semblance of control lies in front of you.

Yes, the doctor is the point person on your team, but fundamentally the responsibility of managing your breathing still lies in your hands. We've covered quite a number of things in the preceding chapters, and hopefully you now have a better idea of what's going on. Most importantly one must understand how the role of the health care team relates to your role in helping yourself.

Just as no two individuals are exactly the same, managing chronic lung disease, or any other chronic disease for that matter, isn't the same for everyone. Perhaps by now a few of the suggestions presented in this book seem relevant and more possible; for instance, beginning an exercise program, following a more advantageous diet or modifying some of those difficult activities of your daily living tasks. First of all, before making any major changes, be sure to discuss them with the doctor.

Adapting to change can be a daunting task, to say the least. Sometimes the sheer magnitude of making a change can be so overwhelming that one never gets started. Fortunately, there are more logical ways to go about it, and the measure of success begins with a plan. Let's take a look at a simple planning process that will be useful in helping you get started in achieving some of those more difficult goals:

1. *Define what it is you wish to accomplish.* Too often frustration evolves from trying to set an unrealistic goal. To set an obtainable goal the desired outcome must be:
   a. **Realistic**: It must be something that is within the realm of the possible. Something that's physically, emotionally and yes, even financially, possible.
   b. **Specific**: Too large of a goal will often not be met. Breaking things down into more workable pieces will enable one to avoid the obstacles that are likely to be encountered.
   c. **Measurable:** It's important to be able to keep track of progress, otherwise it's too easy to get distracted. Losing focus and becoming discouraged are two obstacles to progress.
2. *When does this goal need to be started and completed?* Everything has a timetable, so will your goal. Is there a specific date by which this goal needs to be achieved, or is the timetable more flexible? If a parameter for the completion of the goal isn't set, it's too easy to put it off and not get started or to abandon all efforts before completion.
3. *What steps need to be taken to accomplish this goal?* If the goal is so simple that there is only one step, then the obvious choice is *just do it!* Get rid of the stress of putting things off and get on with it. For everything else that's a bit more involved, a plan is needed. Although the plan may not result in the accomplishment of the goal, if there isn't a plan, there's nothing to fall back on and modify should the need arise. List the necessary steps. There may be only two, or maybe two hundred. Everything begins with a first step. List it, organize it, then get on with it. The better things are thought through, the better the plan will be. The better the plan, the more likely you are to achieve the goal.
4. *What obstacles will be encountered?* If there were no possible obstacles, there'd be no need for a plan, but more than likely there will be a few speed bumps along the way. Before they interrupt any progress, acknowledge them, write them down, then you're ready for the next obvious step, which is
5. *How can I overcome these obstacles?* The obstacles encountered are most likely why that goal could never be reached before. If any of the obstacles are insurmountable, that goal will never be accomplished as understood. Go back to step one and better define the objective. Having a plan to overcome obstacles doesn't guarantee that there won't be any difficulties, but evaluating those obstacles—real or imagined—provides an advantage for successfully overcoming them.

6. *How am I doing? A review of the progress along the way*: A realistic timeline should be set, one that can be be broken down into at least three intervals: near the beginning, near the middle, and at or near the end. Keeping "score" will help you stay on track. The review periods may be days, weeks, or months. Be realistic,

1. What goal do I want to set?
2.   When does this goal need to be started and completed?
Start: Completed:
3. What Steps do I need to take to accomplish this goal?
1.
2.
3.
4. What obstacles will I encounter?
1.
2.
3.
5. How can I overcome these obstacles?
1.
2.
3.
6. How am I doing: Progress report; what's working and what needs correcting
1/4 way evaluation:
1/2 way evaluation:
3/4 way evaluation:
Final evaluation:

Goal-setting worksheet.

though. The longer the timeline, the more likely one is to lose interest and quit.

The worksheet is only a guideline to help one get started, measure progress and improve the chances of ultimately achieving those goals that just seem to be beyond reach. It's not just useful for planning positive health outcomes; one can use it for about anything that seems out of reach. Years ago, a plan developed in this format helped several young men in my Boy Scout Troop achieve the rank of Eagle Scout—a goal that had been eluding them for quite some time. This worksheet is only a suggestion, not a solution. However, if after discussing things with the doctor, you decide to take steps to better manage your breathing problems, I hope this will help—so don't be afraid to try.

To paraphrase Michelangelo (1475–1564), "The danger isn't in setting your goals too high and failing. It's in setting them too low, and being satisfied."

Additional Reading

Susan Ward, 21 January 2020, "Your Guide to Setting Personal and Business Goals," www.thebalancesmb.com.

Glossary

Accessory Muscles of Ventilation: Any of the muscles recruited to increase ventilation when breathing is labored, including the sternocleidomastoids, scalene and pectorals minor muscles.

Acid/Base Balance: (medical) A mechanism developed by the body to keep bodily fluids as close to a neutral pH as possible, i.e., neither too acidic nor alkaline.

Acids: Substances that yield hydrogen ions and/or accept shared electrons from a base. The ph is less than 7.0.

Activities Director: A professional involved with inpatient care who consults with other team members to ensure continuity of care.

Acute: Describing a disease process that is of recent onset and anticipated short duration.

Acute Care: Health care where the patient receives active but short-term treatment for injury, illness or recovery from surgical procedures.

Adoptive Cell Therapy: Involves the transfer of cells to a patient that have been modified with the goal of improving immune function. Cells may be from the patient or from a donor.

Adrenergic Receptors: Specific receptors such as epinephrine (adrenaline) that are targets of catecholamine.

Advanced Cardiac Life Support (ACLS): A set of clinical algorithms for the urgent treatment with lifesaving measures.

Aerobic Threshold: The uppermost limit of exercise beyond which the buildup of lactate acid rapidly increases.

Aerobics: Exercises that are performed in the presence of free oxygen.

Aerosolize: To suspend fine solid or liquid particles and mist.

Agonist: A chemical that binds to a receptor and activates the receptor to produce a biological response.

Allergens: Substances capable of inducing allergy or specific hypersensitivity.

Allergic Asthma: Also known as atopic asthma or extrinsic asthma; Caused by particles suspended in the air which cause the airways to narrow and inflame, leading to reversible obstructions.

Allergist: A physician who specializes in the diagnoses and treatment of allergies.

Alpha Adrenergic Receptors: A group of receptors present on cell surfaces of some effectors' organs and tissues that are innervated by the sympathetic nervous system when bound by specific adrenergic agents.

Alpha-1-antitrypsin (AAT): A genetic disorder that may result in lung or liver disease.

Alveoli: Small balloon-like sacks at the end of the bronchioles through which oxygen and carbon dioxide are exchanged.

Anabolic Steroids: Synthetic steroid hormones that resemble testosterone in promoting the growth of muscle.

Anatomy: The branch of biology concerned with the study and structure of organisms and their parts.

Anticholinergic: Of a group of substances that block the action of the neurotransmitter acetylcholine.

Antigenic Drift and Shift: The process in which two or more different strains of a virus combine to form a new sub-type.

Antioxidants: Compounds that inhibit oxidation. Oxidation is a chemical reaction that can produce free radicals that may lead to cellular damage.

Arterial Blood Gas (ABG): Blood drawn from an artery that measures oxygen and carbon dioxide levels as well as the body's acid base (pH) levels.

Aspiration Pneumonia: (medical) Occurs when unwanted contents such as food, drink, saliva or vomit enters the lungs.

Assisted Living Facility: A facility for people with disabilities or for adults who are unable to live independently.

Asthma-COPD Overlap Syndrome (ACOS): An overlap syndrome condition that shares features of at least two or more widely recognized disorders, in this case, asthma and COPD.

Atelectasis: A condition where portions of the lungs collapse partially or completely. The most common complication following surgery.

Atopic Asthma: The most common form of asthma, resulting in inflammation of the airways caused by allergic reactions. Often associated with a genetic connection.

Atypical Pneumonia: Often called "walking pneumonia"; also known as myco-plasma pneumonia. A highly contagious disease easily spread by respiratory droplets and often resulting in mini epidemics.

Autonomic Nervous System: The part of the nervous system responsible for control of bodily functions that are not consciously directed, such as breathing, heartbeat and digestion.

Bacteria: Biological single cells capable of ingesting foods, excreting waste and reproduction. Many are beneficial for life, many are not.

Barometric Pressure: The pressure within the atmosphere of Earth. The sum of all gases present in the atmosphere.

Beta-2 Adrenergic Receptors (B2): Receptors that rapidly respond when stimulated and relax the smooth muscles of the airways.

Bilevel Positive Airway Pressure (BiPAP): Pressure support provided during non-invasive ventilation. Different pressures are used during inspiration and exhalation.

Biologics: Medical products manufactured from or extracted from biological sources.

Black Box Warning: Required by the FDA for certain medicines that carry serious safety risks or other important information.

Blebs: Small collections of air between the lung and outer surface of the lung.

Borg Scale of Perceived Exertion: A subjective scale used to describe the intensity of exercise.

Breath Activated Nebulizer (BAN): A device used with compressed air to convert liquid medicine into a mist to be inhaled into the lungs.

Bronchial Pneumonia: A condition that results in multiple patches of infiltrates in one or both lungs.

Bronchial Spasm: A sudden constriction of the smooth muscles in the walls of the bronchi.

Bronchiectasis (acquired or congenital): A condition in which portions of the descending airways remain persistently widened as a result of loss of elastic tissue and/or smooth muscles of the airways.

Buffers (bases): Chemical compounds that combine with acids in an effort to moderate the pH.

Bulla: Formed when blebs become larger or come together to form a large cyst.

Calorie: A unit of energy needed to raise the temperature of one gram of water one degree centigrade.

Capillaries: The smallest blood vessels in the body that convey blood between the arterial and venous systems.

Carbon Dioxide (CO_2): A gas consisting of a carbon atom and double bonded oxygen atoms. It's formed in respiration and absorbed by plants in photosynthesis.

Carbon Monoxide (CO): A colorless, odorless toxic gas formed as the result of incomplete combustion.

Cardiomegaly: Abnormal enlargement of the heart.

Cartilage: Resilient elastic tissue found in numerous body parts. Not as hard as bone but less flexible than muscle.

Case Manager: A person with administrative responsibility for formulating a coordinated, comprehensive plan for individuals who need post-hospital care or assistance.

Chest Physiotherapy (percussion): Medical intervention to assist the movement of pulmonary secretions from peripheral airways to more central airways to aid expiration of mucus.

Chronic: (medical) A disease or disorder that develops slowly, does not resolve spontaneously and is unlikely to be cured.

Chronic Bronchitis: Condition caused by frequent infections of the bronchi, resulting in a productive cough for at least three months for the past two consecutive years.

Cilia: Fine hair-like projections from cells in the airways that sweep in unison to remove fluids and particles.

Cold Turkey: Abrupt and complete cessation, as of smoking, without supportive medication.

Collagen: The main structural protein found in skin and other connective tissue.

Combined vs. Dissolved Oxygen: "Combined" refers to the oxygen molecules attached to the hemoglobin of the RBC. "Dissolved" refers to oxygen diffused from the alveoli into the liquid portion of the blood that exerts a pressure gradient necessary to assist the oxygen molecule to combine on the RBC.

Complex Carbohydrates: Longer chains of sugars which take longer to digest and cause blood sugar levels to be more stable.

Congestive Heart Failure (CHF): A weakness of the heart that leads to buildup of fluids in the lungs and other body tissues.

Continuous Positive Airway Pressure (CPAP): Supportive pressure applied and maintained non-invasively to the airways to keep airways open and assist ventilation throughout the breathing cycle. Often used to treat sleep apnea.

COPD (Chronic Obstructive Pulmonary Disease): Lung disease that is characterized by airflow obstruction that is not fully reversible. Includes chronic bronchitis and emphysema.

Corticosteroids: A group of natural and synthetic hormones that are used to treat conditions related to allergic reactions.

Cortisol: A hormone produced in the adrenal cortex. It decreases the immune response to various stresses by decreasing pain and swelling.

Covid-19: A member of a large family of viruses named for the bulb-tipped spikes that project from its surface giving it the appearance of a corona or crown. First detected in December 2019 and rapidly spread usually by airborne transmission resulting in a worldwide pandemic.

Cross Protection: The process where antibodies formed when the body is recovering from an infection may offer some immune protection from different but similar agents.

Croup: An infection of the larynx, trachea and bronchial tubes. May be caused by bacteria or a virus and usually affecting children. Inflamed vocal cords produce a harsh barking cough.

Cystic Fibrosis: A hereditary disorder affecting exocrine glands. Causes abnormally thickened mucus which blocks pancreatic ducts, intestines and airways.

Cytokine Storm: A potentially fatal immune reaction when an uncontrolled and excessive amount of inflammatory cytokines are released in response to an infection.

Diaphragm: A dome-shaped muscular partition separating the chest contents from the abdominal contents. Plays a major role in breathing.

Diaphragmatic Breathing: Also known as abdominal or belly breathing. Conscious constriction of the diaphragm, causing the belly to rise during inhalation before chest movement. Decreases work of breathing and helps to strengthen the diaphragm.

Diffusion: Net movement from a region of higher to a region of lower concentrations.

Digestion: The process of breaking down food by mechanical and enzymatic action into substances that can be used by the body.

DLCO (Diffusion Lung Carbon Monoxide): A diagnostic study to measure the residual volume of air remaining in the lungs after a maximal exhalation.

Do Not Resuscitate (DNR): A legal order signed by the patient or designate to allow natural death to occur or limit resuscitation measures.

Dopamine: A hormone and neurotransmitter between nerve cells. Most commonly associated with the brain's pleasure and reward centers.

Dry Powdered Inhaler (DPI): A device used to deliver medication to the lungs in the form of a dry powder.

Durable Medical Equipment (DME): Medical equipment that can withstand repeated use such as wheelchairs or oxygen cylinders.

Durable Power of Attorney: A written legal authorization to represent and act on behalf of an individual who may be unable to make informed decisions concerning their own medical care.

Dyspnea: The uncomfortable sensation or awareness of breathing or needing to breathe.

Edema: A condition of excessive fluid collecting in the tissue. Also known as dropsy.

Effusion (pleural): Buildup of fluid between the layers of tissue that line the lungs and the chest wall cavity.

Elastin: A protein forming the main component of elastic connective tissue.

Electronic Cigarette (e-cigarette): A battery-powered device that aerosolizes nicotine for inhalation. Does not burn tobacco.

Emphysema: A medical condition in which the alveoli of the lungs are damaged and enlarged.

Eosinophilic Asthma: Severe asthma marked by high levels of white blood cells called eosinophils.

Eosinophils: Disease-fighting white blood cells most often increased when multi-cellular parasites, allergic reactions or cancer are present.

Epidemic: A widespread occurrence of an infectious diseases in a community at a particular time.

Epiglottis: A flap of cartilage at the root of the tongue which is depressed when swallowing to cover and protect the opening of the trachea.

Epinephrine (adrenaline): A hormone secreted by the adrenal medulla in response to stress. Constricts blood vessels and elevates the heart rate and dilates the smooth muscles of the airways.

Esophagus: A muscular tube with mucous membranes. A portion of the alimentary system that connects the throat with the stomach.

Essential Nutrients: Nutrients that the body cannot synthesize on its own or produce in sufficient amounts. Substances that are necessary to sustain life.

Etasis: A term indicating a dilation or distension of a hollow organ.

Extrinsic Asthma: An overreaction of the immune system that releases substances to increase inflammation. A common form of asthma, often associated with genetic and environmental exposures.

Fight or Flight: Also known as hyper-arousal in reaction to perceived stress. An informal description of a sympathetic response.

Flexibility: Capable of bending or stretching easily.

Float Test: A method of estimating the amount of medicine available in an MDI that does not have a functional counter.

Food Pyramid: Chart developed by the U.S. Department of Agriculture displaying food groups arranged according to recommended levels of consumption in a healthy diet.

Free Radicals: A reactive atom or group of atoms with one or more unpaired electrons that can damage cells, proteins and DNA by altering their chemical structure.

Fungi: Spore-producing members of the fungus kingdom, which includes molds, rusts, mildews, mushrooms and yeasts.

Gastroenteritis: Inflammation of the stomach and intestines from either bacteria or a virus. Causes nausea, vomiting and diarrhea.

GERDS (Gastroesophageal Reflux Disease): A condition in which the esophagus becomes irritated due to acid backing up from the stomach.

Germs: A microorganism that produces disease. May be viral, bacterial, fungal or protozoan.

Glutamate: A neurotransmitter of the brain. It's normally involved in learning and memory.

Goblet Cells: Column-shaped cells found in the respiratory and intestinal tract which secrete mucus.

Granulomas: A collection of immune cells that form to wall off substances the body perceives as foreign but is unable to eliminate.

Hemoglobin: A protein containing iron which is responsible for transporting oxygen and carbon dioxide in the blood.

High-Flow Cannula: An oxygen supply system capable of administering up to 100% oxygen which may be heated and humidified in flow rates up to 60 liters per minute. May be heated or cool.

Histamine: A compound that is released in response to injury as well as allergic or inflammatory reactions. Causes constriction of smooth muscles and dilatation of capillaries.

Hospice: Health care that focuses on palliative (comfort) care for the terminally ill patient as well as attending to their emotional and spiritual needs.

Hospitalist: A dedicated inpatient physician who works exclusively in a hospital setting.

Humidity The concentration of water vapor in the air.

Hygiene Hypothesis Theory: A theory that suggests a young child's environment can be too clean to effectively challenge the child's developing immune systems.

Hyperactive-Airway Disease: An informal term used to describe asthmatic conditions with reactive airways in response to stimuli that should not elicit a strong response.

Hyperinflation: A medical condition in which the lungs are abnormally distended.

Hyperventilation: Breathing at an abnormally rapid rate or volume, resulting in excessive loss of carbon dioxide.

Hypostatic Pneumonia: An infection resulting from collection of fluid in gravity-dependent portions of the lungs due to decreased ventilation in these areas and failure to drain bronchial secretions. More often occurring in patients who are bedridden or are unable to cough or deep-breathe.

Idiopathic: Relating to any disease or condition which arises spontaneously for which the cause is unknown.

Immunoglobulin E (IgE): A reactive protein produced by the immune system in response to the presence of a foreign substance (antigen). IgE antibodies recognize and latch on to the antigen in order to eliminate it.

In Case of Emergency (ICE): Recommended cell phone Contacts entry (under the name "ICE") including the name and number of the person one wishes to be called in the event of an emergency. Police and paramedics are trained to look for this information.

Increased Resistance: The reduced ability of air to flow as affected by changes in the diameter of the airways. May not be a constant resistance.

Influenza: A highly contagious viral respiratory infection often occurring in epidemics.

Informed Consent: Obtaining permission before conducting a health care intervention. It discloses the risk vs. benefits of the procedure as well as alternative therapy.

Insulin: A natural hormone made by the pancreas that controls the level of sugar in the blood. Insulin permits cells to use glucose for energy. Cells cannot use glucose without insulin.

Intensive Care Unit (ICU): A specialty unit in a hospital where patients who are dangerously ill are treated and kept under constant observation.

Interstitial Pneumonia: A disease in which the walls of the alveoli become inflamed which may progress to scarring of the alveoli, resulting in pulmonary fibrosis.

Intrinsic Asthma: A non-allergic, non-seasonal form of asthma that often occurs later in life.

Intubation/Extubation: Intubation is a medical procedure where a tube is placed down the throat between the vocal cords and into the trachea to allow pressurized air to inflate the lungs. Extubation is the removal of that tube.

Iron: An essential mineral necessary for the transport of oxygen via hemoglobin in red blood cells.

Laminar Flow: Air flow that follows a smooth pathway without cross currents.

Laryngitis: An inflammation of the larynx most often caused by a viral infection.

Larynx: A tube-shaped organ that contains the vocal cords and is located between the pharynx (back of throat) and the trachea (windpipe).

Leukotriene: Substances released from mast cells, basophiles and eosinophils, causing airway constriction, inflammation and increased mucus production.

Liquid Oxygen (LOX): Obtained from oxygen found in ambient air by fractional distillation in a cryogenic air separation plant. Cooled to -297 degrees Fahrenheit.

Liters per Minute (LPM): A standard unit of measure of volumetric gas flow under standard conditions.

Living Will: A signed document stating medical or legal decisions that are desired in the event one becomes too ill to make informed decisions oneself.

Lobar Pneumonia: An anatomical classification of pneumonia which involves a large portion of a particular lung lobe. Typically caused by streptococcus pneumoniae.

Lung Mass: A spot or area in the lungs that is more than 1.5 inches in size and may or may not be cancerous.

Macrophages: A type of white blood cell of the immune system that engulfs and digests cellular debris, foreign substances or microbes that may cause harm.

Main Stem Bronchus: The first bronchial branch from the trachea, which becomes the right and left main stem bronchi and further subdivides into the lungs.

Mall-Walkers: A program sponsored by various shopping malls to open the mall proper an hour before retail stores are open for business, allowing for registered patrons to use the mall for walking exercise.

Mast Cells: Migratory cells found in connective tissue that release strong chemicals including histamine that cause itching, swelling and fluid leaking from cells.

Maximum Heart Rate: The estimated maximum number of cardiac cycles based only on age.

Metabolism: The chemical process within a living cell or organism that converts food to energy.

Metered Dose Inhaler (MDI): A device that delivers a specific (measured) amount of medication to the airways.

Methylxanthines: A group of naturally occurring agents present in caffeine and theophyllin that stimulate the heart, relax smooth muscles of the airways and produce dieresis.

Monoclonal Antibody Therapy: Antibodies that are laboratory produced and are engineered to serve as substitute antibodies that can restore or enhance the immune system.

Mucous: Membranes that produce mucus.

Mucus: A slightly gelatinous fluid produced in the lungs and various other systems. Similar-appearing secretions expectorated from the lower lungs are also known by the more specific term "sputum." Those produced only by the respiratory system may also be referred to as phlegm.

Mycoplasma Pneumonia: Atypical pneumonia also known as "walking pneumonia."

Nasal Cannula (regular): A device used to deliver supplemental oxygen via a lightweight tube that splits into two prongs and is placed in the patient's nostrils. Liter flow is typically 1–6 LPM.

Nasal Concha: Shell-shaped structures (also known as turbinate) forming the upper structure of the nasal cavities. They contain mucous membranes and increase the surface area of the cavities, providing rapid warming and humidification of inhaled air.

Neoplasm: A new and abnormal growth of tissue in some part of the body.

Neurotransmitter: A chemical substance that when released at the end of a nerve fiber and crossing the nerve junction causes the transfer of the impulse to another nerve, muscle fiber or some other structure.

Nicotine: A highly addictive chemical found in tobacco plants. All tobacco products contain nicotine.

Nicotine Replacement Therapy (NRT): Products that supply low doses of nicotine as an adjunct to assist with smoking cessation

Nodules (pulmonary): Small (less than 1.2 inches) round or oval-shaped growths in the lungs. Often called "coin lesions."

Non-Productive Cough: A cough stimulus that does not result in expectoration of mucus. May be an undesirable side effect of some medications.

Non-Rebreathing-Mask (NRM): A device used to deliver higher concentrations of supplemental oxygen in emergency situations. A face mask is connected to a reservoir bag which is filled with oxygen. Several one-way valves prevent ambient air entrainment, while a valve between the face mask and reservoir bag allows flow from the reservoir but stops exhalation back into the bag.

Norovirus: A group of viruses which are the most common cause of gastroenteritis, or "stomach flu."

Nursing Home: A facility for the residential care of the elderly or disabled patient, where partial or total care is required.

Obstructive Sleep Apnea (OSA): A sleep disorder marked by pauses in breathing of more than 10 seconds while sleeping. Disturbs restful sleep.

Off-Label: Relating to the prescription of a drug for a condition other than that for which it has been officially approved.

Oncologist: A branch of medicine that deals with the prevention, diagnosis and treatment of cancer.

Oxidation: A chemical reaction involving loss of electrons. Occurs when oxygen combines with molecules in food to produce energy, water and carbon dioxide.

Oxygen (O_2): A colorless, odorless gas and the life-supporting component in air, comprising about 21% of ambient gases.

Oxygen Concentrator: A device that concentrates oxygen from room air by selectively removing nitrogen. The result is an oxygen-rich supply delivered to the patient.

Oxygen Conserver: An oxygen delivery device that only allows oxygen flow during inhalation and terminates the flow during exhalation. A special cannula will have one prong that senses negative pressure during inhalation to release the flow, while the other prong will deliver the flow.

Oxygen Cylinder: A storage vessel either under high pressure as a gas or stored as liquid oxygen in a cryogenic storage tank.

Oxygen Debt: When reaching a state of anaerobic metabolism. Occurs when physical activity exceeds the ability to distribute oxygen at the cellular level sufficiently to keep up with the demands.

Oxyhemoglobin: The oxygen loaded form of hemoglobin.

Pack Years: An estimation used to measure exposure to tobacco. For instance, one pack per day for a year is one pack year. The exposure becomes more significant as the estimation nears 20 pack years.

Pandemic: A disease epidemic that has spread across a large region such as several continents or worldwide.

Parasympathetic: A part of the autonomic nervous system that counterbalances the action of the sympathetic system.

Partial Pressure Carbon Dioxide (PCO_2): That part of the barometric pressure that is contributed by carbon dioxide.

Partial Pressure Oxygen (PO_2): That part of the barometric pressure that is contributed by oxygen.

Partial Rebreathing Mask: A device used to deliver supplemental oxygen. A face mask is connected to a reservoir bag which is filled with oxygen. There are no one-way valves. Ambient air entrainment may occur along the mask and partial exhalation may occur back to the reservoir bag. Rebreathing a small amount of exhaled (CO_2) may stimulate the respiratory drive in certain patients.

Patient Assistant Programs: Programs created by pharmaceutical and medical supply manufacturers to help financially needy patients obtain necessary medicines and supplies.

Peak Flow Meter (PFM): A portable device that measures the velocity of forcefully exhaled air. Used to predict asthmatic attacks as well as monitor response to therapy.

pH: An expression of the acidity or alkalinity of a solution.

Phlegm: Mucus produced by the respiratory system, often expelled by coughing. Sometimes referred to as catarrh.

Phosphodiesterase: An enzyme that degrades the action of sympathetic response. By blocking this reaction, the bronchodilator response will be prolonged.

Physiology: The study of normal functions of living organisms and their parts and how systems work together.

Pleura: Two layers of membranes, one covering the lungs and the other attached to the inner surface of the thoracic cavity.

Pleural Effusion: A buildup of excessive fluid between the moist layers between the lungs and the chest cavity.

Pneumococcal Pneumonia: A bacterial pneumonia caused by streptococcus and the most common pneumonia in adults.

Pneumonia: A lung infection caused by virus or bacteria in which the alveoli are filled with pus or other fluid.

Pressure Gradient: The difference in pressures on either side of a membrane.

Primary Care Doctor: A medical professional who provides primary care for all medical conditions and refers patients to specialists as needed.

Protozoan: Protozoons are single celled organisms that are widely found in nature. They prefer water or other moist environments and are helpful to enrich the soil. Normally they are not much of a problem unless contaminated water or food is consumed. Amoebic dysentery is a concern worldwide but is more common in underdeveloped countries. Malaria, a protozoan parasite, is transmitted by the Anopheles Mosquito, leading to serious complications including death.

Pseudomonas: A gram-negative bacteria that can cause lung infections and is one of the leading causes of hospital-acquired pneumonias in patients with decreased immunity or preexisting lung disease.

Pulmonary Arterial Hypertension (PAH): A type of high blood pressure that affects the arteries in the lungs and the right side of the heart.

Pulmonary Fibrosis: A lung disease in which the lung tissue becomes damaged and scarred, limiting the ability to inhale as well as the lung's exchange of gasses with the blood.

Pulmonary Function Test (PFT): A test to measure the volumes and flows into and out of the lungs.

Pulmonologist: A physician whose specialty focuses on diagnosing and treating diseases of the respiratory system.

Pulse Oximeter (POX): A device that measures the oxygen saturation of arterial blood using a sensor in which small increases in the absorption of light during the systolic pulse are used to calculate the oxygen saturation.

Pursed Lip Breathing (PLB): A technique of exhaling through tightly pressed lips and inhaling through the nose. Creates a slight back pressure to splint the alveoli and airways open to decrease the work of breathing.

Rapid Eye Movement (REM): The deepest, restorative level of sleep characterized by rapid eye movements and the propensity of the sleeper to dream.

Receptor: Chemical structures composed of protein that receive and transmit signals that may be integrated into biological systems.

Red Blood Cell (RBC): The most abundant blood cell. Responsible for transport of oxygen and carbon dioxide to and from tissues.

Rehabilitation Facility: An outpatient facility whose primary purpose is assisting in the rehabilitation of disabled persons.

Remodeling: (medical) A change in the structure of the airway walls as a result of chronic irritation. These changes are more apparent in the mid to smaller airways.

Rescue Meds: Medicines intended to immediately relieve symptoms of severe allergies.

Residual Volume: The volume of air remaining in the lungs after a maximum exhalation.

Respimat: Device known as a soft mist inhaler and used for drug delivery for a limited number of inhaled medicines.

Rest and Digest: A description of the parasympathetic nervous system responsible for controlling homeostasis or the balance of bodily systems.

SARS (Severe Acute Respiratory Syndrome): An illness caused by a coronavirus that may lead to pneumonia and respiratory failure.

Septic: (medical) A severe inflammatory immune response triggered by an infection that may be life-threatening.

Sets and Reps: A term used to describe the number of times an exercise is performed. Reps are the number of times an exercise is repeated in a single cycle, while sets are the number of cycles completed of that particular exercise.

Shunt: (medical) A bypass. A pulmonary shunt occurs when there is normal blood flow to the alveoli but no ventilation for gas exchange with the blood. In this case, blood flow will be **shunted** to other portions of the lung where gas exchange is able to occur.

Simple Carbohydrates (Simple Sugars): Sugars chemically composed of only one or two units as opposed to complex carbohydrates, which contain multiple different sugar units. When ingested they are rapidly absorbed into the blood to increase blood glucose.

Simple Oxygen Mask: A face mask used to deliver supplemental oxygen. Does not include reservoirs or one-way valves to redirect flow.

Sinus Cavities: Connected system of hollow cavities in the skull.

Skilled Nursing Assistant: A certified nursing assistant's (CNA) main role is to provide basic care to patients as well as assist them in daily activities as needed.

Small Volume Nebulizer (SVN): A device used with compressed air to convert liquid medicine into a mist to be inhaled into the lungs. Nebulizing continues during inhalation and exhalation until the liquid is completed. Also known as a jet nebulizer.

Smooth Muscle Fibers: Muscle tissue that contracts without conscious control. The layers or sheets are embedded in the lower airways.

Social Distancing: Measures taken to prevent or reduce the spread of a contagious disease by maintaining a physical distance between people and avoiding gathering together in large groups.

Spirometer: An instrument used to measure the capacity of the lungs.

Spontaneous Breathing: Natural breathing of air into and out of the lungs without assistance to initiate breathing.

Spontaneous Pneumothorax: When part of all of a lung collapses and air becomes trapped between the lung and chest wall. The trapped air prevents the lung from re-expanding and is a life-threatening emergency.

Sputum: Respiratory secretions originating from the lower lungs.

Starches: A carbohydrate consisting of numerous glucose units (polysaccharides).

Streptococcus Pneumonia: A bacterial pneumonia caused by streptococcus and the most common community-acquired pneumonia (CAP) in adults.

Stretch Receptors: (medical) Receptors in the lungs that respond to the rate and volume of lung inflations. Near the endpoint, they initiate what is known as the Hering-Breuer reflex to slow and limit further lung expansion.

Strider: An abnormally high-pitched musical breathing sound. Caused by a partial blockage in the larynx or voice box.

Sub-Acute Nursing Facility: A facility providing comprehensive inpatient care for patients with an acute illness, injury or exacerbation of a disease process.

Subjective Measurement: Measurement that has to do with what people say they experience, such as level of pain, nausea, weakness and shortness of breath.

Super Bug: A pathogenic microorganism and especially a bacterium that has developed a resistance to the medications normally used against it.

Sympathomimetics: A pharmaceutical substance whose action basically coincides with the excitation of the sympathetic nervous system.

Tar: Tar is the common name for the resinous, partially burned particulate matter made by burning tobacco in the act of smoking. Tar is toxic and damages the smoker's lungs over time through various biochemical and mechanical processes.

Target Heart Rate: Estimated optimal number of cardiac cycles based on 60% to 80% of one's maximal predicted heart rate.

Tension Pneumothorax: The accumulation of air under pressure in the pleural space.

Terminal Bronchiole: The last portion of a bronchiole that does not contain alveoli, whose primary function is gas conduction.

Theophylline: A bronchodilator of the methylxanthine class

Thoracentesis: A minimal invasive used to remove excess fluid accumulated in the pleural space.

Thrush: A yeast infection of the mouth or throat. Although yeast is a normal part of the flora of the mouth, an infection may cause a severe sore throat and is characterized by white patches in the mouth.

Trachea: Commonly known as the windpipe. The large tube that delivers air from the upper respiratory tract to the bronchi that branch into the lungs.

Tracheal Rings: Any of the 16–20 C-shaped bands of elastic cartilage which are found as incomplete rings in the anterior portion of the trachea.

Triage Nurse: The ER medical professional who determines the priority of patients' treatment based on the severity of their conditions.

Turbinate: A shell-shaped structure (also known as concha) forming the upper structure of the nasal cavities. They contain mucous membranes and increase the surface area of the cavities, providing rapid warming and humidification of inhaled air.

Turbulence Flow: Movement of a fluid or gas characterized by chaotic changes in pressure and flow velocity.

Upper Respiratory Infection (URI): An infection of the upper part of the respiratory system above the lungs. It may be due to any number of viral or bacterial infections.

Valsalva Maneuver: To forcefully exhale with the nostrils and mouth and glottis closed. This increases the pressure in the middle ear and the chest. The increased pressure in the thoracic cavity reduces the amount of blood flowing into the veins leading to the right atrium of the heart.

Ventilator: A medical device to assist in the process of circulating and exchange of gases in the lungs.

Ventilation Perfusion Mismatch: Also known as a V/Q mismatch. A condition where one or more areas of the lungs receives a disproportionate amount of blood or oxygen flow.

Venturi Mask: Often called a Venti-Mask, a device that allows a precise amount of inspired air to mix with oxygen through a fixed jet. The result is a higher flow of gas with a fixed percentage of oxygen.

Vest (the): An airway clearance device designed to assist patients in the mobilization of retained secretions.

Vial of Life (the): Often referred to as Lifesaving Information for Emergencies (LIFE). A program that allows individuals to have their medical information ready in their home for emergency personnel to reference during an emergency.

Virus: A submicroscopic infectious agent that replicates only inside the living cells of a host organism. They infect all life forms from animals and plants to microorganisms including bacteria.

Visiting Nurse: A nurse who visits and treats patients in their homes.

Vocal Cords: Twin folds of tissue in the throat that are key in creating sounds through vocalization. They are stretched horizontally from front to back across the larynx. They remain open when breathing but vibrate during phonation.

Voice Box: A tube-shaped organ that contains the vocal cords and is located between the pharynx (back of throat) and the trachea (windpipe).

Watchful Waiting: An approach to a medical problem where time is allowed to pass before medical intervention or therapy is used. During this time repeat testing and monitoring is performed.

Wheeze: Also known as sibilant rhonchus. A high-pitched whistling or rattling sound that is the result of partial obstruction of the airways.

Yeast: Single cell microorganisms classified as members of the fungus kingdom. Part of the normal flora of the mouth.

Index

accessory muscles of ventilation 13, 88
Accolate 35
activities of daily living (ADL) 97–101
acupuncture and acupressure therapy 39
acute vs. chronic definitions 16
adrenergic receptors 30; *see also* Alpha and Beta receptors
Advair 35
aerobics defined 20; threshold 123
Aerobid 34
Aerospan 34
agonist, definition 29
Albuterol 31`
allergic vs. hypersensitivity reactions 29
allergy testing and immunotherapy 39
Alpha and Beta receptors 30
Alpha-one Antitrypsin (AAT) 21
alveoli 11, 149, 151, 161–163
Alvesco 34
Aminolophyn 32
anabolic steroids 34
Anoro Ellipta 35–36
anticholinergics 33
antigenic shift 145
antioxidants 38, 110
antitussive cough preparations 38
Arcapta Neohaler 31
Armon Air Respi Clik 34
Arnuity Ellipta 35
arterial blood gas (ABG) 69
Asmanex 35
aspiration 10; aspiration pneumonia 151
asthma: atopic, eosinophilic, extrinsic, intrinsic, overlap syndrome 21–34
atelectasis 156
Atrovent 33
autonomic nervous system 29
Azmacort 35

barometric pressure 13, 70, 72
Beclovent and QVAR 35
Beta-two receptors 30
Bevespi aerosphere 35
bifurcation of trachea 10
black box warning 31
Borg Scale of Perceived Exertion 126
bronchial spasm 22
bronchiectasis 165
bronchitis 16, 161, 168
bronchodilators 29–33
breath activated nebulizer (BAN) 47
BREO Ellipta 35
Brovana 31
buffers (bases) 14

calories 74, 105
capillaries 11
carbohydrates, simple and complex 107–109
carbon dioxide (CO2) 11, 81, 108
cardiomegly 160
cartilage, tracheal 9
chest physiotherapy (CPT) 92, 94; *see also* percussion and PEP therapy
chlorofluorocarbons (CFC) 28, 45
chronic vs. acute bronchitis 17
cilia 10, 169
Cinqair 36
collagen 20; *see also* elastin
combined oxygen 13, 70; *see also* oxyhemoglobin
Combivent 33
concha, nasal 7
congestive heart failure (CHF) 160
COPD and emphysema 17, 18
corticosteroids vs. anabolic steroids 33–35
cough preparations 38
COVID-19 148

CPAP and BiPap 58, 83
croup 23
cytokine storm 149

dextromethorpham 38
diaphragm 13, 87, 90, 110; *see also* pursed lip breathing
diffusion of gasses 11–12, 74, 163–164
digestion 105
dissolved oxygen and carbon dioxide 70–71, 120–123, 125
drug formulary tiers and co-pay 64
dry powder inhaler (DPI) 28, 49
Dulera 35
Dupixent 36
durable medical equipment (DME) 77
dyspnea 68, 88, 124–125, 127

elastin 20; *see also* collagen
emergency evacuation strategies 82–86
emergency room protocols 135–139; *see also* triage nurse
eosinophilic 36
esophagus and epiglottis 9
essential nutrients 106, 109
expectorant 38

Fasenra 36
fats, saturated, trans, mono, polyunsaturated 106–113
fiber, soluble vs. un-soluble 112
flexibility 19, 119–120, 130
float test for MDI 43
Flovent 35
food guide pyramid 106
Foradil 31
fortified foods 106
free radicals 109
fruits and vegetables 109

gastro-esophageal-reflex-disease-syndrome (GERDS) 161
generic medicine 63
germs, bacteria-fungi-protozoa-viruses 141–143
glucose 108
goblet cells 10, 17
guaifenesin 38

hemoglobin 13, 70–71, 168; *see also* oxyhemaglobin
herbal and integrative remedies 38
histamine 33
hospice 138

Hydrofluoroalkane (HFA) 28, 45
hygiene hypothesis theory 24
hyperactive airway disease 21
hyperinflation 19
hyperventilation 20

immunoglobulin antibodies (IgE) 36, 110
Incruse Ellipta 33
influenza 144
informed consent 133
insulin 108
Intal 35
interval training 127
intubation/extubation 137
iron 13, 110

lactose intolerance 111
laryngitis vs. croup 9, 23
larynx 9, 23
leukotriene blockers and mast cell stabilizers 35
lifestyle modifications 39
living will and durable power of attorney 139
long acting bronchodilators (LABD) 31–32

main stem bronchus 10
malnourishment 106
mast cells 33
MaxAir 31
metabolism 105
metered dose inhaler (MDI) 28, 42
methylxanthenes 32
monoclonal antibody therapy (anti IgE therapy) 36
mucus, consistency and color 6, 102

nebulizer, BAN, HFVM, JET, SVN, USN 28, 47
nicotine replacement 171–174
Nucala 36
nutrition facts labels 113

obstructive sleep apnea (OSA) 158
off label use of drugs 37
omega-3 fatty acids 38, 112
oxygen debt-hypoxemia 70, 123
oxygen home devices: concentrators, cylinders, LOX 77–80
oxygen interfaces: cannulas and masks 11, 58, 61 68–69, 75, 81
oxyhemoglobin 70, 120–125; *see also* combined oxygen

partial pressure of oxygen (PO2) and carbon dioxide (PCO2) 70
patient assistance programs 66
peak flow meter (PFM) 51
percussion and PEP therapy 92–94; *see also* chest physiotherapy
performist 31
pH 14; *see also* buffers
phytochemiccals 109
pleurisy and pleural effusion 152–153
pneumonia 151–152
pneumothorax 164
positive expiratory pressure therapy (PEP) 94
Prednisone 34
pressure gradient 13, 70
ProAir 31
proteins 107, 110
Proventil 31
pseudomonas infection 142
Pulmicort 35
pulmonary artery hypertension (PAH) 162
pulmonary edema 164
pulmonary fibrosis 163–164
pulmonary function test (PFT) 26, 41
pulmonary nodules vs. mass 153
pulmonologist 27
pulse oximetry (POX) 70
pursed lip breathing (PLB) 46, 89, 90–91, 188; *see also* diaphragm

receptor 29
red blood cell (RBC) 13, 19, 70–71
remodeling 17
residual volume 19, 26
Respimat soft mist inhaler 28, 43, 48

Seebri Neohaler 33
self assessment 101–103
Serevent 31
simple sugars 108
Singulair 36
sinus cavities 7
smoker's cough 10, 169
smoking cessation medicines 171–172
smoking cessation techniques 173–176
smooth muscle fibers 10
spacer device 43
Spiriva 33
spirometer PFS 26; incentive spirometer 157

starches 108
step therapy for meds 64
Stiolto 33
Stiolto Respimat 35
strength training equipment 128–130
strength training reps/sets 128
strider 23
sub-acute/rehab facilities 137–140
surfactant 156
Symbicort 35
sympathomimetic 29

tai-chi and yoga 39
target heart rate 126
terminal bronchiole 19
Theo-Dur 32
Theoair 32
Theophylline 32
thrush infections 142
Tilade 36
tracheal rings 9
traveling with oxygen 82–84; *see also* oxygen home devices
Trelegy Ellipta 35
triage nurse 135; *see also* emergency room protocols
Tudorza Pressair 31, 33
turbinate, nasal 7
turbulent vs. laminar flow 88

Uniphyl 32
upper respiratory infection (URI) 16, 143
Utibron Neohaler 35

V-Max O2 125
Valsaiva maneuver 129
ventilation/perfusion mismatch 162
ventilators 137
Ventolin 31
The Vest 93; *see also* chest physiotherapy
vitamin C and E 38
vocal cords 9

weather, effects on breathing 72–74
wheeze 22

Xolair 36
Xopenex 31

Yupelri Pro 33

Zyflo 36